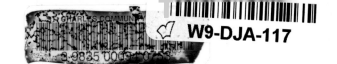

The Long Baby Boom

The Long Baby Boom

An Optimistic Vision for a Graying Generation

JEFF GOLDSMITH

The Johns Hopkins University Press
Baltimore

© 2008 The Johns Hopkins University Press
All rights reserved. Published 2008
Printed in the United States of America on acid-free paper
2 4 6 8 9 7 5 3 1

The Johns Hopkins University Press
2715 North Charles Street
Baltimore, Maryland 21218-4363
www.press.jhu.edu

Library of Congress Cataloging-in-Publication Data

Goldsmith, Jeff Charles.
    The long baby boom : an optimistic vision for a graying generation /
Jeff Goldsmith.
        p. cm.
    Includes bibliographical references and index.
    ISBN-13: 978-0-8018-8851-9 (hardcover : alk. paper)
    ISBN-10: 0-8018-8851-4 (hardcover : alk. paper)
        1. Baby boom generation—United States—Psychology. 2. Baby
boom generation—Retirement—United States. 3. Baby boom
generation—Health and hygiene—United States. 4. Baby boom
generation—United States—Social conditions—21st century.
5. Health attitudes—Age factors—United States. 6. Medical care—
United States—Forecasting. I. Title.
    HQ1063.2.U6G654 2008
    305.2—dc22   2007041649

A catalog record for this book is available from the British Library.

*Special discounts are available for bulk purchases of this book. For more
information, please contact Special Sales at 410-516-6936 or specialsales@
press.jhu.edu.*

The Johns Hopkins University Press uses environmentally friendly
book materials, including recycled text paper that is composed of at
least 30 percent post-consumer waste, whenever possible. All of our
book papers are acid-free, and our jackets and covers are printed on
paper with recycled content.

To my daughter, Amy Goldsmith

Contents

Acknowledgments

I would like to thank several people who helped me with this book. They include Sara Zapolsky and Shereen Remez of AARP; Robert Berenson and Eugene Steuerle of the Urban Institute; Michael Koetting and my son, Trevor Goldsmith, both of the University of Chicago; Dawn Malone and Bonnie Schelor of Bon Secours Health System in Richmond, Virginia; John Bertko of Humana Corporation; Jay Olshansky of the University of Illinois; Jane Boon Pearlstine of New York City; and Stan Amy of New Villages Group in Portland, Oregon. My editor, Wendy Harris, at the Johns Hopkins University Press provided gentle and substantive guidance in revising my manuscript. Anita Gupta, Kelly Cush, and Susan Sleight, all of Charlottesville, provided invaluable research assistance.

Introduction

Fresh from liberating the world from the Axis powers, America's Greatest Generation came home from World War II and brought forth a baby boom. Seventy-six million children emerged from this remarkable postwar celebration, almost four children per family. American society has not been the same since.

The baby boom increased the U.S. population 44 percent in just eighteen years! American society had to re-create itself to accommodate the new arrivals. Each social institution the baby boomers touched, from elementary schools to university to the family and the work world, they fundamentally reshaped, not only by the press of their sheer numbers but also by their unique, high-maintenance approach to the world. At each turn in their lives, baby boomers have torn up the script and started afresh.

Today, the advance guard of this generation's legions is within four years of reaching a bristling societal Maginot Line: age 65. According to many pundits and forecasters, the aging baby boom threatens the U.S. economic future.

Consider the comments of Kotlikoff and Burns in *The Coming Generational Storm:*

> You see a government in desperate trouble. It's raising taxes sky high, drastically cutting retirement and health benefits, slashing defense, education, and other critical spending, and borrowing far beyond its capacity to repay. It's also printing tons of money to "meet" its bills. You see major tax evasion, high and rising rates of inflation, a growing underground economy, a rapidly depreciating currency, and more people exiting than entering the country. You see political instability, un-

employment, labor strikes, high and rising crime rates, record-high interest rates. You see financial markets in ruin. You see America plunging headlong toward third world status.[1]

Consider Charles Mann's assessment in an *Atlantic Monthly* article, "The Coming Death Shortage":

Longevity induced slowdown could make young nations more attractive as investment targets, especially for the cash strapped pension-and-insurance plans in aging countries. The youthful and ambitious may well follow the money to where the action is. If Mexicans and Guatemalans have fewer rich old people blocking their paths, the river of migration may begin to flow in the other direction. In a reverse brain drain, the Chinese Coast Guard might discover half-starved American postgraduates stuffed into the holds of smugglers' ships. Highways out of Tijuana or Nogales might bear road signs telling drivers to watch out for *norteamericano* families running across the blacktop, the children's Hello Kitty backpacks silhouetted against a yellow warning background.[2]

According to the doomsayers, the baby boom generation promises to be a gigantic albatross around society's neck. They expect the next several decades to be a time of social involution in the United States, as boomers cease working, retire to Florida, and cash in their entitlements to social support, shamelessly voting to raise taxes on their children and grandchildren to support their leisure, robbing the country of its future.

As they so often are, the pundits are going to be wrong—about the timing, the impact, and the required remedies. We call these particular pundits "catastropharians"—economists, politicians, and journalists who carry on a proud, masochistic tradition of viewing the American future as one of unavoidable conflict and decay. The catastropharians proffer a doomsday social policy scenario about the coming senior boom and a "take your castor oil" agenda of "painful but necessary" changes in our social programs to avert fiscal Armageddon.

While no one knows for certain what will happen in the next twenty years, the multiple, bleak assumptions underlying this grim scenario have not been carefully examined. Catastropharians simply *assume* that baby boomers will follow their parents' and grandparents' life paths, as well as mimic their political values. They assume that longer life-spans will translate into lengthier periods of unproductive and parasitic activity on the part of older Americans. Then they superimpose this behavior on the structure of our current entitlement programs, which they assume will not adapt meaningfully to the pressures, and tote up the damage. The future will thus unfold, with past as prologue, and demography as destiny.

What's Wrong with This Picture?

As this book demonstrates, the catastropharian thesis is riddled with flaws. The vision of the baby boomers as a gigantic societal albatross is a myth in the making. Not only are the catastropharians wrong about the next twenty years. Their social prescriptions are also the wrong medicine for American society. They offer a static, zero-sum vision for what is, in fact, a dynamic, growing and creative economy and society. The crisis they envision is eminently avoidable, not by the politically untenable solutions they offer, but rather by listening to the generation itself and helping its members do what they say they intend to do.

American society does face a crisis, but not the one envisioned by catastropharians: a crisis of meaning for a new generation of older Americans for whom retirement makes neither economic nor human sense. The "golden years" vision of retirement as an extended, dry-land version of a luxury cruise is a failed social experiment (and one of relatively recent vintage). Many boomers who observed their parents' and grandparents' lengthy drift at the end of life have made a fundamentally different life plan.

Most baby boomers will probably not retire in the conventional sense. According to multiple AARP surveys, most baby boomers do not plan on ceasing to work at 65, as their parents did. Some 80 percent of baby boomers plan on working past age 65, with a plurality of boomers doing so because they enjoy working rather than because they need the money. (Now you understand the reason why the word *retired* no longer appears in AARP's name.)

For some boomers, continuing to work will be a sad necessity, because millions currently lack the private pension coverage or savings to support themselves if they are not working. For millions more boomers, however, retirement simply will not be a satisfying life path. Indeed, 84 percent of workers older than age 45 plan on continuing to work "even if they are set for life." Boomers will remain taxpayers and part of the active economy far longer than most economists assume. It is likely that millions of boomers will be income-producing assets, not liabilities, on society's balance sheet well into their 70s and beyond.

Moreover, we cannot replace the boomers if they do wish to retire. The United States faces a looming and potentially crippling shortage of skilled workers that affects our vital infrastructure—schools, the health care system, government at all levels, and even manufacturing. The baby bust, which bottomed in 1975, has created a huge hole in the midcareer skilled U.S. work force. Forecasts suggest a looming and costly shortage of skilled workers in the next decade, a shortage that deepens further in the decade that follows. Knowledge-based enterprises will have a particularly difficult time replacing their older workers.

While boomers will not be able to fill all these gaps, personnel policies that push older workers out of the skilled positions in our economy will be forcefully reexamined in the next few years. In some segments of our work force, the cost of replacing experienced older workers could exceed the increased expenses related to retaining them. Rather than encouraging boomers to retire, we need to revise our tax and pension policies, as well as the Social Security and Medicare programs, to encourage boomers to remain engaged, productive (and taxpaying) citizens.

Healthier Aging: An Emerging Reality

The link between aging and illness also requires reexamination. Age 65 will define neither the end of work nor the beginning of serious illness. Indeed, thanks to steady improvements in the health status of so-called elderly people, age 65 will come to be viewed in the

near future as a late middle age biologically, rather than old age. Because age 65 is a gateway to the Medicare program, however, pundits
have carelessly assumed some correlation between eligibility for public benefits and the onset of illness.

The health status of people older than 65 has improved steadily
over the past two decades, not merely in the United States but in
most Western countries. Kenneth Manton, at Duke University, estimated the pace of reduction in morbidity at 1.5 percent per year for
the past twenty years (a trend that has accelerated over the period).
These health improvements among older Americans mean that far
fewer will be institutionalized and that many will be able to work
longer and enjoy a more balanced and active independent life than
their parents or grandparents did.

Longer working lives and more active life-styles will, in turn, translate into improved health, both physical and mental, for millions of
older Americans. Even as they reach the age of 60, boomers typically
think of themselves as seven years younger than their chronological
age. Hardly a single member of this generation identifies himself or
herself as "elderly." That label is reserved for those who have reached
age 78. Of course, this does not mean that the generation will live or
work forever, but those experts predicting some cataclysmic social
event when baby boomers turn 65 are destined to be disappointed.

Starting Over

To assess the likely trajectory of the baby boom generation over
the next twenty years and what it means for reshaping social policy
toward older Americans, this book explores the baby boomers' current state: their lives, health, and wealth and how they differ from the
generations of older Americans that preceded them. It considers the
baby boomers' present plans, their diverse values and life circumstances, and their political outlook and attachment to the political
process.

It also assesses the future contributions of older workers, considers what is being done to encourage longer and more diverse work
roles, and explores the health status of baby boomers and the threats

that chronic illness poses to their independence and earning capacity. To provide additional context, the book frames the legacy social programs put in place four generations ago to respond to the crisis of the Great Depression and discusses how those programs have come to dominate our present federal government.

Next, the book outlines a rational social policy response to the evolving needs of baby boomers. This discussion necessarily encompasses strategies for the needed redesign of public programs such as Medicare and Social Security, as well as tax and employment policies for older Americans, to take account of baby boomers' distinctive circumstances and needs.

Finally, it returns to the issue of the diverse circumstances of baby boomers, and what can be done to assure a just and humane response to those who are likely to struggle with the next twenty years.

A Jujitsu Approach to Social Policy

In some forms of martial arts, such as aikido or jujitsu, the secret of defeating a larger opponent is to capitalize on his momentum to move him in a direction you want him to go. Much discussion of "entitlement reform" deals generically with older Americans without focusing on the specific values and needs of this generation. There is already momentum in the revealed preferences of the baby boom generation toward activity and independence, healthier aging, the creation of new enterprises, a more "virtual" work life, and a better balance between work and leisure. Figuring out how to encourage and capitalize on this momentum is the secret of a win-win social policy toward the coming senior boom.

Optimism about our society's future is currently out of fashion in U.S. cultural and intellectual circles. World-weary pessimism and cynicism about our collective incapacity to "face reality" and "make the tough choices" is the dominant tone of social commentators, policy analysts, and their patrons in the political world. Gregg Easterbrook discusses the anomalous contrast between this pessimism and our nation's extraordinary economic and social record in his book *The Progress Paradox: How Life Gets Better While People Feel Worse.*[3]

Not surprisingly, pessimism and cynicism have not produced many solutions, merely a lot of patronizing caricatures and unworkable ideas, as well as a sense that Americans are chronically overmatched by the big social challenges. Because the generation is so vast, fully one-quarter of American society, it has functioned as a gigantic Rorschach blot onto which a generation of elders—politicians, editorial writers, and novelists—has projected their neuroses and anxieties. Because they fundamentally misunderstand the plans and values of baby boomers and project onto them not only their anxieties but also the political agendas of their parents and grandparents, the prophets of doom have lost connection with the very people who must support vitally needed societal changes.

There is an urgent need to change the conversation about the baby boom and its future. The expensive script written for baby boomers' next twenty years, like all the other generational life scripts written for them, is destined for the trash heap. Baby boomers, even the less-fortunate ones, are fundamentally optimistic about their *own* futures. Most boomers haven't spent fifteen minutes thinking about how Social Security or Medicare will actually affect them, for the obvious reason that they do not consider themselves "old." How they approach these topics will likely be shaped by their personal experiences over the next twenty years, not by some ironclad historical logic or the opinions or values of their elders.

This is an optimistic book about a generation of optimists, an unintentional but strategic irony. If we were start from scratch, given what we know about the needs and values of this difficult generation, we would not build the structure of public programs and work roles that we have inherited from our terrifying brush with societal collapse during the Great Depression. We would also not be catastropharians.

This book asks the question, If you were designing a social policy that fit baby boomers' attitudes, values, and dreams, what would it look like? What the United States and its citizens urgently need is a pro-work, health-promoting social policy that aims to keep baby boomers (and those who come after them) healthy, engaged, and contributing. This book offers a vision of what that policy might look like.

The Long Baby Boom

Prologue

Robert Smallwood (February 2011)

Robert Smallwood looked out from the redwood deck of his home at the sun rising over Mount Rainier and the Seattle skyline. The air was crystalline and cold. It was a rare, completely sunny winter day on Bainbridge Island, Washington. A gentle murmur rose from the rocky beach below. Smallwood had finished reading the online version of the Sunday *New York Times* on his computer, and he was enjoying a large, steaming fresh mocha on a comfortable deck chair.

Reading the Sunday paper was one of his rare, calendar-marking rituals—it reminded him that it was, in fact, a weekend. It had been nearly a decade since he had worked in an office, when his workweek was demarcated into five days on and two days off. Smallwood retired in 2002 from his position as an executive in a large, prosperous nonprofit hospital system in Seattle, where he was responsible for new business development. Smallwood had had a successful career in health care management. The new enterprises he created, in partnership with the system's physicians, now generated $200 million in revenues and 62 percent of the $2 billion organization's operating profits.

Three days ago, Smallwood had turned 64, and he celebrated by taking a long kayak excursion around the island with his wife, Irene, and cooking a lovely dinner at home. His wife, who was 62, worked as a teacher in a local, alternative elementary school and was a passionate environmental activist and organic gardener. She was also a member of the County Board of Supervisors and engaged in the intensely personal business of local Democratic Party politics.

Smallwood had not ceased working at age 55; rather, like more than a few of his colleagues, he became a self-employed "free agent." In 2002 Smallwood morphed into a new, self-directed role: mentor, angel investor, and business adviser to a younger generation of entrepreneurs in his chosen field. The work was exciting, stimulating, and rewarding, both intellectually and financially.

So far, six of these new ventures had sputtered along on fitful capital infusions from various private and institutional sources. Four had failed outright. However, two had flowered into large, self-sustaining businesses, multiplying his initial small six-figure investments thirtyfold. Collectively, these new businesses employed 2,100 people, scattered all over the West. Smallwood, who had about $3 million in retirement funds when he "retired," now had a net worth of $16 million, not counting his homes on Bainbridge and in Sedona, Arizona, where he went when the sodden Seattle winters became unbearable.

Smallwood, who never had to work again, continued working nonetheless, more or less seven days a week, perhaps three hours a day. Given his modest fixed costs—no mortgage or other debts, Medicare subsidized health care, and a nice stream of cash flow from his 401(k) plan and private investment portfolio, Smallwood had achieved the financial equivalent of a geostationary earth orbit. With just the tiniest bit of push, he could sustain his position as long as he wished to and his health and energy would permit.

"Work" consisted of a more or less continuous broadband Internet connection to a network of many hundreds of professional colleagues scattered around Seattle, the country, and abroad. He was also connected to a bubbling pot of financial and medical news, to the "blogosphere," as well as to a continuous flow of financial reports and executive summaries of his companies. Though he occasionally hopped the ferry over to Seattle and flew somewhere for a professional conference or board meeting of one of his companies, most of his business activity was conducted by spontaneous and scheduled on-line video teleconferences.

Smallwood did miss the water cooler and after-work microbrews with his office colleagues, but he was far better informed now than when he was working. Always somewhat reclusive, he found that his asynchronous networking (sometimes at 1:30 in the morning) offset some of the physical isolation of his largely virtual working role.

His father and mother had retired from factory and nursing jobs, respectively, at the prescribed retirement age of 65. They died, largely of boredom, only eight years later, only three weeks apart, in their condominium in Mesa, Arizona. Traditional retirement simply wasn't going to work for him. Smallwood mused that he could continue what he was doing easily for another twenty years without tiring of it, and he hoped that his good health and energy would enable him to do it.

Peter Porter (September 2007)

It was the night before school started, and Peter Porter felt the same mixture of apprehension and excitement he had felt, an unimaginable fifty-two years earlier, on his first day of school. Porter was doing something few grownups, other than the 1970s television sitcom character Gabe Kotter, had ever done: returning to his old elementary school as a teacher.

Porter had been hired to teach seventh- and eighth-grade Spanish by Meriwether Lewis School in Spokane, Washington, whose principal was scrambling to replace almost half of the faculty that had retired in just three years time. Porter even received a $10,000 signing bonus, a convention Porter thought was reserved for professional quarterbacks and bond traders.

In the late 1950s, Porter had attended Meriwether Lewis as a student. He was a quiet, studious, and gravely serious child, burdened with what he thought were absurd parental expectations. Porter was to be a doctor, and his parents, both busy professionals, had planned out his entire life for him, down to the month. Porter himself wanted to be an astronomer, and he studied the stars with his telescope almost every summer evening. By age nine, he could name three dozen constellations and identify hundreds of stars.

As he ran the gauntlet of high school and college, however, his parents' plans and his own faded into insignificance. Lost emotionally, Porter succumbed to adolescent angst and depression, dropped out of college after two years, and became a lumberjack. He moved to a tiny town in the eastern Washington Cascades and bought a cabin in the woods.

Twelve years of brutal and dangerous physical labor followed, and a solitary, rustic existence in the woods. Like many of his fellow loggers, Porter destroyed his lower back setting choke chains, and he nearly lost his left arm when a huge branch fell on him from a height of eighty feet. As a result, he was in nearly constant pain. Always thrifty, Porter saved thousands of dollars, as his living costs were less than $300 a month. He made a few friends among his fellow loggers, hunting deer and elk with them on weekends during hunting season. Female companionship eluded him, however, and he was often intensely lonely. Porter succumbed to a deepening depression, finding solace on the wet and cold winter evenings in bourbon and occasional poker games with his male friends.

Finally, at age 32, Porter decided that he could manage the physical pain and isolation no longer. He sold his cabin in the woods for about what he paid for it and moved to the university town of Pullman, Washington. He enrolled in Washington State University, majoring in Spanish and agricultural science. On graduation, he moved back to Spokane and found a job with the county agricultural extension service. He also volunteered with a local nonprofit organization that provided help to the large Mexican migrant worker population that worked in the orchards and farms around Spokane.

In 1985 Porter met a young real estate salesperson named Arlene Edwards, who was on her way to being the top residential sales producer in her large real estate agency. They moved in together and then married a year later. Four years later, the Porters had a daughter, Amanda. The relationship and new family prospered, and with their combined earnings, the 1990s real estate boom, and a modest inheritance from Arlene's parents, the couple accumulated sufficient wealth that they were both able to retire in 1999 and focus their attention on Amanda, by then a budding competitive swimmer.

Porter also cultivated his hobby of repairing and showing vintage and classic cars, as well as tutoring community college students in Spanish and trading stocks on the Internet. He traveled to antique and classic car shows around the mountain states. As he advanced into his 50s, however, Porter's depression returned. He also struggled with dependency on painkillers, which he needed for chronic and unremitting back pain, an unhappy legacy of his logging days.

In 2000 the bursting of the dot.com bubble devastated the Porters' investment portfolio, which had been imprudently invested heavily in speculative stocks. To meet margin calls, the Porters had been forced to sell several investment properties at unfavorable prices. What seemed like a comfortable multimillion-dollar asset cushion that could have stretched thirty years all of a sudden receded into the low six figures. Though it still generated enough income to meet the Porters' modest current needs, it fell far short of adequate for the long haul.

Finding affordable health insurance was also a problem, as their local Blue Cross plan rates almost tripled in a six-year period. Retirement did not sit well with the couple, who fought frequently with each other and with their teenage daughter. By late 2005, Arlene had "unretired," returning to her real estate office part-time, and Peter began exploring how to use his skills to earn a current income.

Porter did not wish to return to his position with the county, but he enjoyed using his Spanish, and when he learned that the Spokane public school system faced a catastrophic shortage of teachers and had loosened its credentialing requirements for language teachers, Porter went and obtained his teaching certificate and applied for a position teaching in his old elementary school. The job brought with it not only an income but also generous health insurance and retirement benefits after only ten years. It seemed oddly comforting to be returning to an elementary school that had not materially changed since Porter had graduated from it in 1964.

The prospect of more than thirty years of retirement paled after only six years, and the uncertainties inherent in amateur investing and tensions of an unaccustomed idleness has caused both Porters to return to work. It would take many years to rebuild their asset position, pay for Amanda's college, and find the right balance between work and leisure for the remainder of their lives.

Avril Sanchez (April 2007)

Avril Sanchez sat on the patio of her parents' Riverside condominium and wondered where she was going to find the money for the knee replacement she needed. It hurt to walk, and she was not able to work in her present condition. In late 2005 Avril and her younger sister, Clarita, both unemployed, inherited their parents' condominium free of mortgage when her father passed away. A small, two-bedroom unit, the condo was the only real asset left in their parents' small estate, which had been stripped of its liquid assets by enormous combined medical bills.

The sisters grew up in West Los Angeles, the daughters of a grocery store owner who immigrated to the United States in the early 1950s from Monterrey, Mexico. Her parents worked eighty hours a week building their grocery business, and they pressed both their children to work and study hard. Avril was a tall, slim brunette with enormous brown eyes and a wild, adventurous streak. She did well in school, but by 15, she was hanging out with her friends on the Sunset Strip, entering clubs with false IDs, and flirting with men fifteen years her senior.

Avril was intelligent and, despite the partying, got excellent high school grades. After graduating from high school, she was given a full scholarship to attend prestigious Pomona College. She found suburban Claremont boring and smoggy, and she missed her wild friends in the Hollywood Hills, commuting into town frequently on school nights in a battered MG to continue living the high life.

After two years, she quit college and, in a successful effort to horrify her parents, moved to Las Vegas and became a dancer at the Tropicana. There she met a succession of high-roller boyfriends, who paid her rent and living expenses and took her on holiday to Mexico and the Caribbean.

In her early 30s, Avril broke up with her boyfriend, then overdosed on barbiturates, and was rescued by a paramedic. She entered rehab, where she detoxed and spent the next five months regaining her bearings.

The hospital stay saved her life. Avril gave up drinking and drugs and, with her parents' help, returned to college at California State Northridge, where she finished her B.A. and began training as a laboratory technician. She was hired by the Northridge Hospital in the clinical laboratory and became one of the steadiest and most reliable hospital employees.

However, health problems clouded her work career and life. She developed a deepening depression and withdrew from her colleagues and co-workers. She also began gaining weight, which appalled her. The men who had swarmed around her like moths around a flame through her 20s deserted her in her late 30s and early 40s, as had many of her friends who married and had families to attend to. Her depression affected Avril's ability to work, and she eventually lost her hospital job due to poor attendance. Lacking savings, Avril drifted into part-time clerical employment, keeping a neat and modest apartment in Pacoima, a down-at-the-heels part of the San Fernando Valley.

Her sporadic income enabled Avril to obtain coverage under California's Medi-Cal program, which paid the cost of her antidepressants and an increasing array of drugs for various escalating medical problems. She developed the symptoms of diabetes, for which she required daily doses of insulin, as well as immobilizing back and knee problems. Avril was unaware that she was eligible for disability coverage under Social Security and therefore Medicare, because she incorrectly believed these programs were available only to older people.

Nevertheless, with the depression under control, Avril regained some of her emotional balance. She began doing yoga every morning and began working part time in a small clinical laboratory. Because they could not offer her health insurance coverage, however, the physicians operating the clinic paid her in cash to avoid disqualifying her for Medicaid coverage, on which she had become totally dependent. To lose her Medicaid coverage would have left her completely exposed to the cost of a $1,200 a month medication bill. To remain insured, Avril had joined the underground economy.

As they reached their late 70s, Avril's parents were under siege from their own medical bills and could no longer help her financially.

Her father was partially paralyzed from a catastrophic stroke, and her mother, disabled by arthritis, was unable to care for him. Her sister, Clarita, a nurse, was caring for their parents nearly full time, draining their substantial retirement savings to pay the portion of their chronic care costs not covered by Medicare. By the time they both passed away, their estate had dwindled to $24,000 and the Riverside condo, which the sisters now jointly owned.

Avril and Clarita moved in together and began supporting each other. Their joint income was sufficient to pay for the maintenance and utilities on the condo, car insurance, food, and little else. The $24,000 disappeared quickly.

By 2007, six years shy of eligibility for Medicare and facing limited Social Security checks due to sporadic lifetime employment, the sisters wondered how they were going to make ends meet for the balance of their lives. While Avril has achieved some inner peace, she worries every day how to manage the material side of her life.

All three of these fictional characters are baby boomers, yet their circumstances, needs, and options differ dramatically. They represent three distinct trajectories into the last third of life, which form the basis of a typology that recurs later in this book. This typology is used to test the impact of social policy solutions to the problems likely to arise as baby boomers move through the next twenty years. In the penultimate chapter, this typology resurfaces to help clarify the unique challenges posed particularly by the least-fortunate group.

Those who think of the baby boom as monolithic routinely underestimate the dramatic differences in life circumstances within this generation. This point becomes crucial later in the book, because policy solutions that do not encompass this diversity may well do more harm than good. Even the most skilled forecasting exercise cannot hope to narrow all the potential uncertainties facing the baby boom generation, let alone the broader society. Still, we know enough about the current circumstances of baby boomers to assess those uncertainties and respond to them creatively.

one

The Baby Boom

The Self-Involved Glacier

Recovering from the Great Depression and fighting World War II focused American society's attention elsewhere than on its young people. During the Depression, each American family generated 2.1 births, barely a replacement level of fertility. The ensuing war finally spurred the economy, but it separated families and created uncertainty about the future. Societies experiencing such crises do not create many children: couples without children postpone forming families, while families with children concentrate on feeding and sheltering the ones they already have.

The baby boom generation, in contrast, was conceived in optimism—the euphoric aftermath of global triumph over the Axis powers. Though the rise of the Soviet Union cast a shadow over this triumph, the menacing uncertainty of World War II gave way to a U.S. economic rebirth with seemingly limitless possibilities for its young families. Returning veterans reunited with their spouses, returned to school, and began making babies at a furious pace. During the baby boom, Americans' fertility rate increased to an astounding 3.8 births per family and resulted in a 44 percent increase in the U.S. population (figure 1.1).

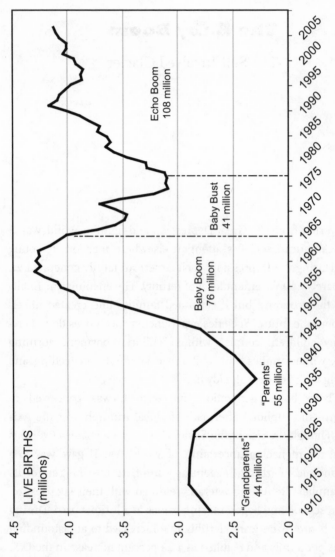

Figure 1.1. The U.S. postwar baby boom
Source: Data from U.S. Census Bureau.

Straining Capacity

The new American family and its needs became the central preoccupation of not only merchants and advertisers but also the popular culture and society. As the baby boom unfolded, the United States was confronted with a massive, rolling capacity problem: how to feed, house, educate, and eventually employ 76 million new people. Making room for the baby boom proved to be a major economic and domestic policy challenge in the years following World War II.

The expansion of elementary education became the most pressing item on the agenda of local government. About 45 percent of all existing public schools were built between 1950 and 1969.[1] In the 1960s and 1970s, America's higher educational institutions, public and private, had to execute a similar dramatic expansion to handle the flood of students. Between 1960 and 1980, the number of college students more than quadrupled, from 2.9 million to 12.4 million.[2] This expansion was not merely a matter of many more people of college age but also a marked increase in their participation rate.

The proportion of baby boomers who graduated from college was far higher than that of their parents' generation.[3] As late as the 1940s, only 5 percent of the U.S. population aged 25 or older had attained a bachelor's degree or higher; only 25 percent had graduated from high school![4] By 1980 high school graduation rates had risen to 67 percent, and 27 percent of the baby boomers went on to achieve a bachelor's degree or higher. From 1940 to 1990, the number of college graduates in the United States grew almost tenfold, from 3.4 million to 32.3 million.[5] This higher educational level has had important implications for baby boomers, and, as will be later discussed, it will influence how effectively they manage their health risks as they age.

As baby boomers graduated, they flooded the labor market with an unprecedented number of people with college or advanced degrees. Baby boomers became the shock troops for a new, knowledge-based economy. Two long economic expansions, interrupted by economic troubles from 1973 to 1981, provided the working capital to fund the expansion of the U.S. work force to accommodate the baby boom generation.

The last phase of this economic expansion was accomplished in the face of a sudden quintupling of energy prices in the wake of the 1973 Arab oil embargo. After a pullback in energy prices in the mid-1970s, there was a less vertiginous but still significant energy price increase in the wake of the Iranian Islamic revolution at the end of the decade. The onset of the Iran-Iraq War in 1980 pushed oil prices to a 2005 equivalent price of more than $100 a barrel and gasoline prices to more than $3.50 a gallon.[6]

For the economy to absorb these two huge energy price shocks and nevertheless create 34 million new jobs in twenty years stands as perhaps the most significant unacknowledged economic miracle of the late twentieth century. Of course, what enabled this miracle was the fact that the baby boom generation itself created explosive growth in demand for every product and service you could think of: real estate and automobiles, household appliances and clothing, computers and electronic gadgets. In turn, this new demand created the jobs that employed the people consuming the products. The remarkable U.S. economic growth in the 1980s and 1990s was "powered by boomers."

Dominating Popular Culture

The baby boom ruthlessly monopolized American popular culture. Baby boomers (and their young parents) became the first mass market for the emerging American television industry. Television shaped the popular images that held boomers mesmerized in their childhood and adolescence, as well as created a mass retail market for new consumer products. The television-viewing audience, with only 4.4 million people owning television sets in 1950, grew to 50 million in one explosive decade.[7]

Tens of millions of Americans, children and parents, watched the *Lone Ranger* and *Superman, Captain Kangaroo* and the *Mickey Mouse Club,* and *Rocky and Bullwinkle.* They experienced the siege of the Alamo and bought Davy Crockett faux coonskin caps; attended Disney's animated full-length feature films, such as *Cinderella, Sleeping Beauty,* and *101 Dalmatians;* and visited Disney's theme parks. Television also introduced to boomers a new generation of musical performers, future pop culture icons such as Elvis Presley and the Beatles. These new stars catalyzed the growth of a modern entertainment industry, whose stars commanded the attention of the world's youth. Interestingly, the highest-grossing rock music acts in 2005–2006 were all either boomers themselves, such as Madonna and U2, or older musicians, such as Eric Clapton, Paul McCartney, and the Rolling Stones, whom boomers had listened to in their teens and twenties.[8]

The new Interstate Highway System, whose construction began in 1955, enabled baby boomers to become the most mobile and geographically liberated generation of Americans. Not only did the Interstate system enable rapid intercity movement but it also provided the transportation framework for an astonishing expansion of suburban housing, enabling the boomers' parents to relocate by the millions to the suburbs and yet remain accessible to the city for work and leisure. Cars became central to baby boomers' lives, particularly as adolescents and young adults. Baby boomers grew up in their family cars and, as they aged, they took advantage of markedly improved physical access to explore their country.

The Interstate Highway System not only catalyzed economic growth and enabled the emergence of dispersed employment sites but also enabled a cosmopolitan, restless, and highly mobile generation of young Americans. No longer confined to a city neighborhood or a town, as their parents and grandparents had been, baby boomers were able to experience the breadth and diversity of the vast American continent.

Steeped in Politics

Political consciousness and activism shaped the values of this enormous and influential generation. Baby boomers grew up in the shadow of nuclear holocaust, hostages to the terrifying nuclear standoff between the United States and the Soviet Union. To characterize it as a "cold war" does not do justice to its psychic impact. Baby boomers learned at an early age that they and their families could literally be vaporized in a sudden firestorm of atomic war. They were taught to cower under their school desks in "duck and cover" drills, as well as to listen for the high-pitched whine of a Civil Defense alert on their transistor radios, which could signal the end of the world.

Seeking social justice for the oppressed was central to the baby boom political agenda.[9] Older baby boomers heard John Kennedy's stirring call to action in his 1961 inaugural address: "Ask not what your country can do for you. Ask what you can do for your country." The boomers' older brothers and sisters initiated political protests over civil rights, particularly voting rights, access to public education, and freedom from discrimination in the workplace for black Americans. This activism gave rise to a mass political movement and forced the Johnson administration and Congress to intervene and guarantee voting rights and access to education for minorities. This movement shortly produced a welter of new federal programs to attack both rural and urban poverty. As Leonard Steinhorn argued in his 2006 book, *The Greater Generation,* baby boomers have not been sufficiently credited for their role in fostering a commitment to social justice.

Though some of its leaders, such as Betty Friedan and Gloria Steinem, were older, baby boom women were the foot soldiers of the women's movement, which demanded and secured women's rights in the workplace, family, and society at large. By redefining women's priorities to encompass careers and the freedom to decide when or whether to have children, this feminist revolution fundamentally reshaped the American workplace and family.

Baby boom women also catalyzed a revolution in women's health, symbolized by the publication in 1970 of *Our Bodies, Ourselves,* a book that encouraged women to reshape the health services they used to meet their own and their children's needs, rather than simply to obey the health care system's dictates.[10] The feminist revolution thus gave rise to a consumer movement in health care, which helped level the sharp gradient in power and knowledge between patients and their physicians.

Unfortunately, the baby boom also represented a demographic resource for politicians—a massive cohort of military-aged young people that swelled U.S. military power. Dramatic escalation of the

Vietnam conflict came in 1965, the year in which, by grisly coincidence, the leading edge of the baby boom generation reached military age. This unpopular war against a resourceful enemy killed more than 58,000 young Americans—boomers and their older brothers and sisters (compared to about 3,300 dead in the first four years of the U.S. expedition in Iraq). More than 3 million soldiers rotated through Vietnam during the thirteen-year-long war, and more than 300,000 brought home injuries that scarred them for life.[11]

The Vietnam War altered the life course and shaped the political values of an entire generation of young men. Every male boomer born before 1957 was touched in some way by the military draft and the prospect of being sent to Vietnam. Between 50,000 and 100,000 young Americans fled to Canada to avoid the draft.[12] Millions of others hid out in college or graduate school, intentionally crafted shelters from the draft, or in public service jobs that brought them draft deferments.

The Cultural Tyranny of the 1960s

As the first baby boomers reached their teens in the mid-1960s, the United States experienced a surge of violent crime (figure 1.2) and an even more shocking wave of mass urban violence in its largest cities; Detroit, Chicago, Los Angeles, and Newark experienced the most extensive damage. Some of the cities that went up in flames during the middle 1960s, such as Detroit and Newark, have never recovered.

The nation's divorce rate also surged in the 1960s (figure 1.3), coincident with the baby boom's reaching the age of family formation. This sharp generational discontinuity had far-ranging implications for the shape of the American family and for the lives of baby boomers' children, an increasing proportion of whom lived in one-parent families. A surge in children born out of wedlock paralleled this trend. The disintegration of the nuclear family and rising crime and violence contributed to a sense that U.S. society was unraveling before our eyes. A wave of political controversy and recrimination ensued, which is, remarkably, still going on some forty years later.

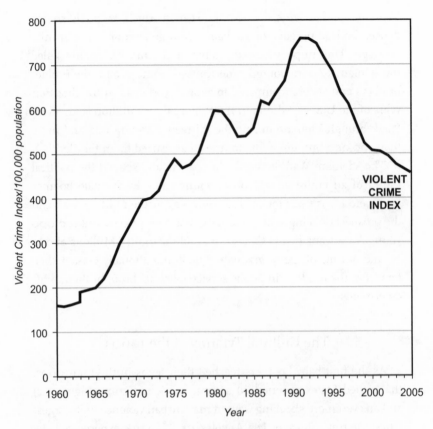

Figure 1.2. U.S. violent crime index, 1960–2005
Source: Data from FBI Uniform Crime Reports.

Americans are still angrily debating what happened during the
1960s. The rising crime and divorce rates, as well as rising births out
of wedlock, were cited by conservative social critics as signposts of
cultural decadence and moral decline.[13] The 1960s were not a
uniquely American cultural phenomenon. Other countries, notably
France, Germany, and China, experienced wrenching cultural up-
heaval during the same period, fired by the coming of age of a large
generation of postwar children.

Everyone in American society experienced the turbulence of the
baby boomers' adolescence whether they wished to or not—initially
their parents and grandparents and now, in an unwelcome cultural

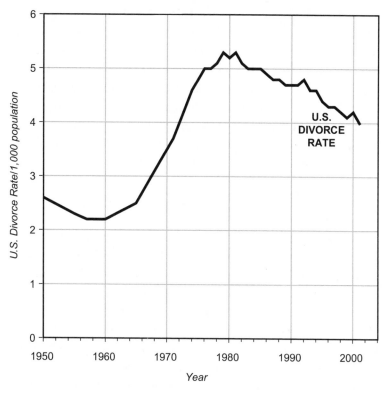

Figure 1.3. U.S. divorce rate, 1950–2001
Source: Data from U.S. Census Bureau.

echo, baby boomers' own children. Many Generation X'ers, who were born between 1965 and 1990, resent the cultural tyranny of the 1960s and the grip boomers seem to have on the cultural imagination. Paul Begala, a former aide in the Clinton White House and now a television pundit, once referred to the baby boom generation as "a giant garbage scow." In the definitive novel that coined the term "Generation X," Douglas Coupland inveighed against self-involved boomer parents, whose children toiled in what he called McJobs that led nowhere, while increased costs of living made it impossible for them to live independently.[14]

An irritating assumption by social observers of the baby boom is the unvoiced belief that the baby boomers were then and are today culturally and politically homogeneous. This is manifestly false. Not every boomer protested against the Vietnam War or against the oppression of minorities or discrimination against women. Indeed, even today, baby boomers split fifty-fifty on whether entering the Vietnam War was a mistake and whether losing it was merely a failure of national will.[15] The political reaction to the Vietnam War and the darkening of American culture split the society, including boomers themselves, and created a cultural division that has become, even with the passage of four decades, the principal "values" cleavage in U.S. politics.

Suspicious of Power

Baby boomers grew up suspicious of political power. The most enduring and pervasive political attitude of boomers for more than thirty years has been the high level of mistrust of politicians and institutions. Political attitudes of baby boomers' parents were shaped in the crucible of the Great Depression and World War II. Memories of a successful societal mobilization against the Depression and defeat of a frightening global military foe left in boomers' parents the residue of strong faith in U.S. political institutions.

Political values of baby boomers, on the other hand, were forged in a climate of disillusionment and mistrust. The Vietnam conflict had a personal effect on virtually every male boomer who is currently older than 50 and on his younger brothers and sisters indirectly. Vietnam, a war expanded stealthily by Lyndon Johnson and lengthened furtively by Richard Nixon, permanently colored attitudes toward governmental authority and truthfulness. This suspicion finds powerful echoes in the widespread unpopularity of the war in Iraq.

The Watergate crisis, which drove President Richard Nixon from office, further reinforced baby boomers' beliefs that political power served merely its own ends and is reliably abused. Only 32 percent of boomers surveyed in 2004—thirty long years after Watergate—believed that government "will do what is right most of the time."[16]

These two events—the Vietnam War and Watergate—had a powerful catalytic effect on boomers' political attitudes. Division over the Vietnam War and the backlash against the civil rights and abortion

rights movements not only split baby boomers but also shattered the
Democrats' New Deal coalition, separating many working-class whites,
Catholics, and southerners from the party. Beginning in 1976, a succession of presidential candidates of both political parties successfully
campaigned, directly or indirectly, against the federal government.
This culminated in President Clinton's remarkable (and insincere)
pronouncement in his 1996 State of the Union address that the "era of
big government is over."

It is impressive how durable baby boomers' mistrust of government has been. In 1970 public opinion surveys found that a minuscule 3 percent of boomers were "very confident" in statements made
by government leaders. With the benefit of thirty years' experience,
the proportion of boomers surveyed in 2002 who said they were
highly confident in the veracity of government statements grew to a
whopping 6 percent. Boomers highly confident in Congress actually
fell (from 16% to 13%) in the ensuing thirty years.

Mistrust of politicians and politics may be responsible for changing voter participation patterns as baby boomers entered the political
system. Two major changes in political participation coincided with
baby boomers' becoming enfranchised: the emergence of a large bloc
of so-called independent voters, and the decline in voter participation
rates (figure 1.4). Both of these trends accelerated markedly after

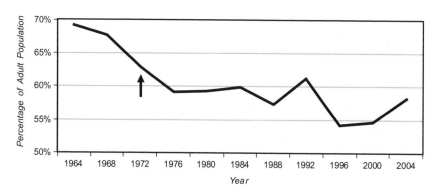

Figure 1.4. Voter participation, 1964–2004
Source: Data from U.S. Census Bureau.

1971, when the Twenty-sixth Amendment to the U.S. Constitution lowered the voting age from 21 to 18.

Today, independent voters outnumber members of either political party. Independent voters and nonvoters together comprise a majority of the voting-age U.S. population. How the nonaligned voters behave determines in large measure which major party's candidates prevail in state or national elections (figure 1.5).

Baby boomers are the core of a large and resource-rich pool of potential supporters for future third-party presidential candidates and potentially a third political party. In a 2004 poll taken for AARP, 56 percent of boomers said they believed the country needs a strong third party, compared to 37 percent of their parents' generation.[17] The same survey found that 16 percent of baby boomers were not registered to vote, double the number of their parents' or grandparents' generation.

Boomers mistrust concentrated power of all kinds, not merely political institutions. They are truly the children of Thomas Jefferson. Only 22 percent of baby boomers surveyed in 2002 expressed a great deal of confidence in corporate leaders, 20 percent in those running colleges and universities, and 13 percent in leaders of organized religion.[18] Since the 1970s, confidence by baby boomers rose in only two institutions: the military and, remarkably, the executive branch. Because Richard Nixon had been president in the early 1970s, the modest rise in trust in the executive branch is at least somewhat comprehensible. This has almost certainly dissipated in the past five years owing to widespread disillusionment over the war in Iraq and rising hostility to the Bush presidency. The end of the military draft may have elevated baby boomers' esteem of this once feared institution.

Boomers' suspicion of power has been institutionalized in a strong investigative press, both print and television. Courageous investigative reporters unearthed the Pentagon Papers and drove the hated Richard Nixon from office. The Internet has unleashed a new generation of resourceful freelance journalists, the bloggers, upon the wealthy and powerful. A major impact of an aggressively populist digital, broadcast, and print media has been to reinforce the public's belief that power and wealth corrupt those who possess them.

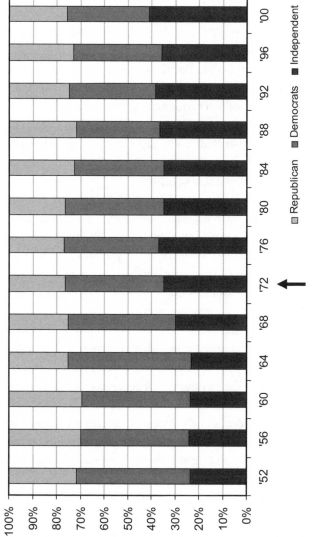

Figure 1.5. Increase in independent voters, 1952–2000
Source: Data from the National Election Studies, 1948–2002 National Election
Studies Cumulative Data File.

Personal Optimism: The Defining Character Trait of Baby Boomers

The disjunction between personal optimism and profound cynicism about the political system is a striking feature of baby boomer attitudes. If you were to crystallize a single defining character trait of baby boomers, it would be optimism about their personal lives. In a 2003 survey, 67 percent of older boomers and 80 percent of younger boomers believed that their lives would be better in five years, compared to only 37 percent of older Americans.[19] Only 5 percent of older boomers and 1 percent of younger boomers believed their lives would be worse in five years than today. The fact that most baby boomers have experienced only one serious recession in their adult lifetime (1979–81) may have fostered this optimism.

Baby boomers have already outdistanced their parents economically. On average, they have achieved higher incomes and accumulated more wealth.[20] However, as they usually do, these averages conceal significant disparities. While the top 20 percent of the boomers have a median net worth of $766,000, the bottom 20 percent have a median net worth of only about $1,500. Almost 7 percent of boomer households have zero or negative net worth.[21]

Despite this disparity of life circumstances and despite the turmoil of the Iraq war and post-9/11 uncertainties about our security, an extraordinary 82 percent of baby boomers surveyed in 2004 professed a great deal of satisfaction with the way things are going in their lives (including a remarkable 68% of those with household incomes below $25,000 per year). Sixty-nine percent of baby boomers strongly agreed with the statement, "What happens to me in the future mostly depends on me," and a comparable percentage agreed with the statement, "When I really want to do something, I usually find a way to succeed at it."[22]

For someone to reach the age of 50 with a faith in his or her personal future and power to achieve personal goals largely unimpaired by personal experience is a remarkable testimony to an almost genetically based optimism (as well as the durability of U.S. economic growth). This sunny optimism seems to be a uniquely American trait, which irritates many European colleagues and friends.

The anomalous contrast between an almost religious faith in the boundless possibilities of their personal futures and a deep-seated mistrust of society's major institutions complicates the task of political leadership. Baby boomers' personal comfort with optimism seems to have influenced their choice of presidents. After an unhappy experience with the dour and gloomy Jimmy Carter, Americans have rewarded with second presidential terms three leaders (Reagan, Clinton, and George W. Bush) who, despite profound differences in their stated political agendas, mirrored that sunny boomer optimism and faith in the future.

This pervasive suspicion by baby boomers of government could well spell an end to so-called entitlement politics, with its plantation-style reliance of large voting blocs on powerful political patrons. Baby boomers might not be willing to raise taxes to fund government-sponsored benefits for themselves in coming years. Because a large enough proportion of baby boomers will still be working or depending on passive income, many would see a tax increase as hurting their own pocketbooks.

As earlier discussed, boomer disillusionment with the political process has materially weakened both political parties, which have both struggled to find a way of communicating not only with boomers, but with even more disillusioned younger voters. Profound differences in life circumstances and needs within the baby boom generation may complicate efforts to find a unified political theme that engages all boomers.

Boomers who have bombproof retirement funding and plentiful financial assets and home equity will most likely have much less interest in government "safety net" programs for the "elderly" than those who have no resources and compromised health status. This latter group, however, may contain a larger number of voters who have already disengaged from the political process and thus do not vote to express their economic interests.

Of course, political attitudes will probably change as these issues become less theoretical and more immediate. AARP research found that faith by boomers in the solidity of Social Security and Medicare increased somewhat in the 1998–2003 period, perhaps conditioned somewhat by the 2001 tech stock crash and advancing age of the older boomers. However, only 54 percent of boomers surveyed in 2003 were "very or somewhat confident that Social Security will be available for them when they retire," and 47 percent were "very or somewhat confident" about Medicare availability.[23]

It is worth remembering that the younger half of the boomers are solidly "midcareer" (e.g., in their 40s) and "old age" is still a long way off, both biologically and emotionally. Fifty-something boomers do not identify with their elders or do not think of themselves as "old." Rather, 63 percent of them feel younger than their actual age.[24]

Tracking changes in baby boomers' political attitudes as they age will be a major preoccupation for pollsters and political scientists for the next several decades. However, that single-issue entitlement politics focused on protecting New Deal social guarantees will excite the same reflexive passions and loyalties among boomers as it did among their parents and grandparents is difficult to imagine, given what we now know about baby boomers' attitudes toward government and political leaders.

To assess how baby boomers will respond to the social safety net will require us to understand the political and economic promises made to an earlier generation of older Americans. It will help as well to appreciate how different the twenty-first-century U.S. economy and society are from that scary world of the 1930s, when so much of America's promise almost blew away in a prairie dust storm. Much of the controversy over the economic impact of the aging of the baby boom stems from how boomers will interact with the "legacy" programs of the New Deal. That controversy is explicated in greater detail in the following chapters, along with some of the major flaws in the catastropharian thesis.

two

The Social Safety Net for Older Americans

The Expensive Legacy of the New Deal

Understanding how the aging members of the baby boom generation will interact with the New Deal–Great Society social programs is vitally important, not only to their own futures but also to the future of the U.S. economy. Even at this late date, however, there are more questions than answers. Other than those who have wrestled with these programs as advocates for their parents, baby boomers have thought little about Social Security and Medicare, primarily because they do not think of themselves as old. To comprehend why the boomer experience with these programs is likely to be so different from that of previous generations, a brief history lesson is required.

The present social safety net for older Americans—Social Security and Medicare—was the legacy of an unimaginably painful economic tragedy, the Great Depression of the 1930s. Almost four generations have passed since this tragedy, and the social contract that emerged from it must be seen in the sociopolitical context that gave rise to it.

In the first decades of the twentieth century, the U.S. economy was in the midst of a historic transition from an agrarian to a manufacturing economy (the transition currently under way in China). Farming represented half of the U.S. economy of 1930, and almost 21 percent of the population worked in farming.[1] The agrarian era in the United States ended suddenly and catastrophically—in a thunderous and terrifying collapse in commodity prices, credit, and land values during the early 1930s.[2]

From 1929 to 1933, the gross domestic product of the U.S. economy shrank by more than 30 percent.[3] As the Depression deepened in the 1930s, one-quarter of the U.S. work force was idled. Credit collapsed, asset and consumer prices plummeted, and, in a sickening chain reaction, 5,000 banks and 90,000 businesses failed.[4] Millions of elderly (as well as nonelderly) Americans found their assets disappearing into a black hole of cascading bank failures, and many lost their homes and farms to foreclosure.

Farm-raised children had already begun migrating to the city, where the new jobs were, during the first two decades of the twentieth century, leaving their parents and grandparents behind in the towns where they grew up. As a consequence, a disproportionate number of the nation's older citizens lived in rural areas and depended on the suddenly decimated farm economy. They kept their savings in passbook accounts in banks that failed, and they bought and worked their farms on credit that suddenly disappeared.

By the time the Depression bottomed in the mid-1930s, half of all older Americans were on locally financed relief rolls. Male life expectancy was only 58 years in 1930.[5] In addition, only 19 percent of those age 25 or older were even high school graduates, and only 4 percent had graduated from college.[6] Health status was fragile, and the health care system functioned almost completely on a cash-on-the-barrelhead basis.

An Expanded Federal Role in the Economy

The Depression constituted an authentic national emergency. Roosevelt responded to that emergency with a remarkable and durable expansion of the role of the federal government in the private economy and society. Institution by institution, banking first, then farming, then income security, Roosevelt and the Congress rebuilt shattered U.S. economic infrastructure. Federal deposit insurance guaranteed the safety of savings, restoring confidence in the nation's battered banks and creating a stream of fresh deposits. New regulations and a new agency, the Securities and Exchange Commission, governed public securities markets, assuring a higher standard of transparency and disclosure for financial transactions. New public credit temporarily replaced vanished private credit for farms and small businesses.

The most visible piece of the New Deal, however, was Social Security, a payroll-tax-financed universal pension plan enacted in 1935. Social Security replaced a discredited and inadequate patchwork system of state pensions and local relief programs. It also contained a raft of programmatic initiatives for nonelderly people, including unemployment insurance, child welfare, maternal child health services, and the like.[7]

Not everyone was covered by Social Security; in its initial form, 9 million workers were excluded from coverage for diverse reasons.[8] Poor (mostly black) migrant workers and sharecroppers, domestic help, and people working in small businesses such as grocery stores and soda fountains were left out. Also excluded were railway workers and workers in state and local governments, which had their own pension systems.

Neither Roosevelt nor Congress intended the "thin safety net" of Social Security to provide the sum total of retirement security for American workers. Social Security needed to be supplemented by private pension and retirement guarantees, as well as health benefits (which the government was unable to provide) to be truly comprehensive.

Despite estrangement between Roosevelt and organized labor in the early years of the New Deal, labor unions became an important core constituency of the administration's efforts. Roosevelt and his congressional allies enacted labor laws that protected unions' right to organize workers. New Deal architects worked in tandem with union leaders to assure that benefits guaranteed by the government for the old and the poor were matched in the private sector by corporate guarantees for the working population, extracted from employers through collective bargaining.

With the previously noted exceptions, most employers and employees contributed to Social Security, and the employees began receiving

Social Security benefits at age 65. This age of eligibility was based on prevailing retirement ages in the few private pension systems in existence in 1935 and, more important, the thirty state old-age pension systems then in operation.[9] In the United States, the eligibility age chosen for Social Security was seven years older than the average male life expectancy as of 1930.

To this first generation of older beneficiaries, Social Security was a huge gift. Enacted in 1935, the program began paying benefits only five years later. Indeed, it took thirty years until workers contributed an entire working lifetime of payroll taxes before collecting their promised benefits. For the vast majority of these early beneficiaries, Social Security payments constituted the totality of their income.

The difference between their contributions and the benefits early Social Security recipients received represented a direct, federally managed income transfer to older people from younger workers. Concern about this issue prompted Congress in 1939 to expand eligibility for Social Security to younger people by adding benefits for widows and dependent and surviving children of deceased beneficiaries.[10] A disability benefit for younger workers was added in 1950, further diversifying the generational base of the program.[11]

The Safety Net Extended

Older Americans rewarded Franklin Roosevelt's Democratic Party with overwhelming and unquestioned support. The partnership between Roosevelt and the labor-union movement also had powerful and enduring political consequences. It made the Democratic Party the "party of labor." This linkage survives today, even as labor struggles to find its way in the New Economy.

The New Deal dampened the very real potential for armed insurrection in the nation's devastated rural areas and largely halted the growth of the Communist Party.[12] Roosevelt's activism also forestalled more radical schemes to redistribute wealth, such as the Townsend Plan, and stole the political thunder and constituents of radical populists such as Huey Long and Father Coughlin, the nation's first radio televangelist.

Roosevelt was unable to create a federally guaranteed health benefit as part of the New Deal. Efforts to complement the income security guarantees of Social Security with guaranteed medical coverage faltered in the Truman administration. The powerful American Medical Association and employer groups played a role in opposing what was termed "socialized medicine." As a consequence, it was to be thirty years before Congress would enact federally funded health coverage for older Americans.

In 1965, in the wake of the assassination of President John Kennedy, President Lyndon Johnson pushed through amendments to the Social Security Act that provided universal, publicly funded medical coverage for older Americans. The Medicare program provided coverage for hospital and physician services. Almost as an afterthought, Congress provided coverage for medical services for young families on welfare through the Medicaid program. (In 2007 this legislative "afterthought" cost $336 billion a year split between the federal government and the states.)[13]

The hospital services portion of Medicare was financed as Social Security was, with a payroll tax deduction. The physician coverage portion of Medicare was financed by general tax revenues and "premium contributions" after people reached age 65 and became Medicare beneficiaries. This tax is typically deducted from the beneficiary's Social Security check every month. Medicaid was financed by federal and state cost sharing, both from general tax revenues.

Working in concert with a growing post–World War II national economy, the Social Security system including Medicare played a pivotal role in lifting senior citizens out of poverty. The percentage of older Americans living in poverty fell steadily for the next forty years.

Elder Power and Entitlement Politics

At the time Social Security was enacted, the United States was a young country. Only 8 percent of the population was over 65 years old, compared with 12.4 percent today. (At the beginning of the twentieth century, it was even younger, with only 4 percent of the population over 65.) When Social Security was enacted, there were an amazing forty-two working-age Americans available to subsidize re-tirement coverage for every older person. With the advent of the baby boom, the country got even younger, reaching a median age of only 28 in 1964, the final year of the baby boom.

As the baby boom gave way to the baby bust, however, the origi-nally entitled older population emerged as one of the nation's most influential and best-organized political interest groups. According to a Pew Foundation analysis, people older than 50 are twice as likely to be "regular voters" as people aged 18–19 and three times as likely to be registered to vote.[14] (An astonishing 40% of the younger group of Americans are not even *registered* to vote.)

The political constituency for financing Social Security and Medicare benefits was broad-based and powerful: congressional ad-vocates, such as the late Representative Claude Pepper and Senator Ted Kennedy; a new interest group, the American Association of Re-tired Persons (now known as AARP); and a newly powerful lobbying complex of hospitals, physicians, nursing homes, and others who benefited from Medicare payment. Many in government and the pol-icy world believe AARP, with its 36 million members, to be the most powerful interest group in Washington.

Gaps in the Safety Net

In the past thirty years, the parts of our economy that have grown most rapidly, particularly services and retail trade, were those in which benefits costs were low and union representation of workers often nonexistent. Labor markets flooded by the baby boom also be-came a buyers' market, depressing wages as well as enabling em-ployers to offer skimpy benefits to younger workers. According to Peter Capelli, an economist at the Wharton School of the University of Pennsylvania, the flood of workers depressed hourly wages of pro-duction workers by an inflation-adjusted 15 percent from the 1970s to mid-1990s.[15]

Skimpy benefits fit the short-term needs of both the employer and the employee. After all, how much does a teenager or person in his or her 20s care about retirement funding? And how much do young people, who tend not to become sick (and are, as is well known, immortal), care about health insurance? As a consequence, the New Deal public-private safety net of retirement security and benefits guarantees developed increasingly spacious cracks through which tens of millions of American workers have fallen.

Over the years, many not-so-young Americans fell through the cracks as well. The population lacking health coverage (which may include workers in low-wage industries, self-employed individuals, younger widows or divorced women, recent immigrants, and those who retire or lose their jobs before age 65 without retirement benefits)[16] is not only diffuse and fragmented but also unorganized politically, especially compared to the focused constituencies that benefit from entitlements aimed at older people. Indeed, they have little in common with one another but the lack of private health and pension coverage.

Some social observers have suggested that by electing to protect only the most vulnerable populations (the elderly through Social Security and Medicare, the poor through welfare and Medicaid), the New Deal–Great Society programs may unintentionally have weakened political support for universal health coverage that would have benefited the society more broadly.[17] Advocates for the poor and for older Americans have proved far more vigorous in defending their own entitlements than in expending political capital on behalf of the uncovered.

Entitlement Politics for the Baby Boomers?

Our political system has responded slowly and fitfully to this growing coverage gap. Because they tend to vote in smaller proportions than the wealthy or those currently receiving entitlements, uncovered populations, including, most important, young people in transition from home to autonomous adulthood, have not presented an attractive political constituency for those who advocate extending benefits on their behalf.

The political logic of the New Deal was straightforward: the party that confers public benefits on a group can count on its votes going forward. A Democratic president champions voting rights for black Americans; ergo blacks will vote Democratic in the future. Republicans regularly propose significant tax cuts on the wealthy; ergo wealthy taxpayers will vote Republican.

Whether baby boomers will follow this political logic appears questionable. Recent AARP surveys have confirmed the thinness of baby boomers' commitment to entitlements: "Although they are more liberal on certain moral and social issues than their predecessors and expect a lot of things from government, this does not necessarily translate into support for social welfare programs or traditional entitlements. Boomers are less likely than [their elders] to favor welfare programs for lower-income people and far more likely to support privatizing Social Security and Medicare."[18]

While it may be premature to sound the death knell for entitlement politics, the baby boom generation is likely to turn a basilisk's eye toward any politician promising fresh entitlements. In a 2007 Democracy Poll survey, when asked if the federal government would spend new money wisely or waste it, 84 percent of likely voters aged 50–64 said the money would be wasted. (Imagine what the unlikely voters think?)[19] About half of the baby boomers surveyed recently by the AARP do not believe that they will receive benefits from Social Security and Medicare comparable to those received by their parents and grandparents, though the degree of confidence in these programs rose somewhat (from abysmally low levels) from 1998 to 2004.[20]

The Unpromising Political Calculus of Entitlement Reform

The New Deal–Great Society legacy has become, in economic terms, the principal business of the federal government. Medicare, the federal portion of Medicaid, and Social Security collectively account for about 40 percent of the current federal budget, compared with 30 percent in 1986.[21]

Unlike defense and education, which must receive congressional funding annually, spending for these three programs rises automatically as the number of people eligible to receive them grows. Social

Security payments are set by formula, not by annual appropriation, and grow apace with wages. Payments to hospitals, physicians, nursing homes, and other providers of care are also set by formula and basically grow as the volume of services increases.[22]

Entitlement programs to support older Americans have both tremendous political rigidity and economic momentum, because they commit the federal government and taxpayers to huge future expenditures unless the formulae, eligibility standards, or, heaven forfend, the promised benefits themselves are altered. The spending formulae for paying for medical services are, as I argue later, highly inflationary, because they provide lucrative incentives to health care providers to maximize their patients' use of health care regardless of their needs.

I previously explained why older people are such a formidable political force. In the next twenty-five years, the number of claimants on guaranteed social benefits will grow dramatically. Between 2011 and 2030, 76 million baby boomers will reach the statutory age of entitlement, which will vary between ages 66 and 67, depending on the age of the beneficiary.[23] They bear down on this venerable benefit threshold like a glacier. Because the principal solutions to the problem seem so unpalatable politically, the glacial pace of demographic change makes dithering, posturing, and denial by policy makers and politicians virtually inevitable.

Entitlement Politics Works for Health Care Providers

A major reason for the political reluctance to reform these programs is that older Americans are not the only people "entitled" by the New Deal–Great Society legacy programs. Medicare has become an entitlement program for providers of health care. Payment under these programs amounts to almost half of the income of the nation's hospitals and well more than half of the livelihoods of many surgical and medical specialists.

Under the present health payment ground rules, health care providers have powerful economic incentives to increase federal spending, because the more care they render to the Medicare population, the more they earn. Medicare and Medicaid payment functions much like a taxi meter—except when the driver throws the flag, he or she drives you where he thinks you need to go, and someone else (e.g., the taxpayer) pays the fare.

Medicare and Medicaid became the growth engine for the U.S. health economy, a colossus that, by itself, is roughly the size of the entire German economy.[24] In 2007 Americans will spend almost $2.3 trillion on health care, of which 34.5 percent comes from the Great Society health-financing programs.[25]

Tinkering with the formulae that pay for medical care through these programs is, effectively, tinkering with the blood supply of a powerful and hungry creature. Changing how health care providers are paid also feeds the insecurities of the largest and best-organized bloc of American voters. I talk in greater detail about why these programs are broken and how to fix them in chapter 6 on Medicare.

A Fiscal Train Wreck?

Catastropharians, such as former treasury secretary Peter Peterson, former Fed chairman Alan Greenspan, and public sector economists such as Laurence Kotlikoff, believe that unchecked entitlement spending will destroy the U.S. economy. In a recent study, Kotlikoff and Burns argue that when you roll the existing structure of social obligations for Medicare, Medicaid, Social Security, and other federal and state income-transfer programs forward fifty years, bake in fifty years of presumably uninterrupted health cost inflation, and superimpose a much larger population of entitled older people, you arrive at a $72 trillion present-value estimate of future promises.[26]

Of this amount, promised Social Security benefits constitute $22 trillion and Medicare and other health- and income-security programs another $50 trillion. To put this in perspective, the present U.S. GDP is more than $13 trillion. So the tab for future social spending for baby boomers and their children, *if we assume current ground rules,* amounts to almost six times the current total wealth generated by the U.S. economy in a year.

According to Eugene Steuerle of the Urban Institute, expected lifetime benefits paid out to people upon retirement by these two pro-

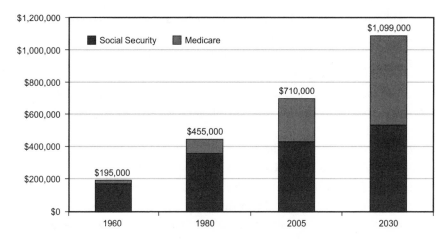

Figure 2.1. Social Security and expected Medicare benefits for average-wage
two-earner couple
Source: Urban Institute, Washington, D.C., 2005.

grams have soared, particularly as the cost of Medicare has risen. According to the Urban Institute, lifetime payouts for an average two-
income couple ($36,600 each) rose from $455,000 in 1980 to
$710,000 in 2005 (in 2005 dollars). This is expected to rise to almost
$1.1 million for a couple reaching eligibility in 2030. Most of the in-
crease is in the Medicare portion of the benefit, highlighting the part
of the program in which the most fiscal risk resides (see figure 2.1).

According to Kotlikoff and Burns, the fiscal burden of sustaining
these payouts is worsened by the effect of increases in the so-called
dependency ratio, the ratio of those "entitled" older people to the
younger "working" population that must fund, through taxes and
payroll deductions, this substantial future benefits obligation. The ratio of beneficiaries to younger taxpayers was far lower when Social
Security and Medicare were enacted.

The catastropharian argument is, in a nutshell, that the larger financial obligations of an older population, when spread over a
smaller base of younger workers, will create a ruinous fiscal overhang for society, an enormous claim on the income and resources of
its younger citizens. The catastropharians further argue that because
we already shortchange the young by underfinancing both education

and health care for children, fiscal and political pressure to fund entitlement spending for older people will further aggravate this imbalance and create the potential for explosive intergenerational conflict over limited societal resources.

Of course, this is, at its core, a *political* argument concealed in a fancy econometric model. As Kotlikoff and Burns point out, politicians often rely on economists for "creative writing"—inventing sophisticated econometric rationalizations for their political positions.[27]

It is absurd to argue that our political system is going to tolerate sustained hyperinflation in health care costs for fifty years without doing anything. It is equally absurd to argue that there will be no change in our net tax burden given the cyclical character of budget deficits, state and federal. Experience has shown that deficits have a marvelous way of concentrating policy makers' attention on out-of-control spending.

Who Subsidizes Whom?

Despite the political gloss that these programs are "insurance" programs funded entirely by the beneficiaries themselves, Social Security and Medicare are, in fact, a massive, federally managed income transfer from younger workers to older people, retired or working.[28] These programs transfer wealth from renters who cannot afford to buy homes to older people, 80 percent of whom own their own homes (the majority of which are free of mortgages). Though most of them do not realize it, young people working in fast-food franchises who lack both health insurance and pensions are funding social benefits to retired doctors and lawyers who are eligible for benefits by virtue of their age.[29]

This income transfer is a feature inherent in social insurance mechanisms generally. That is not inherently a bad thing. Advocates of the New Deal–Great Society programs have argued that these intergenerational subsidies contribute to social solidarity.[30] It is worth reminding ourselves that the vast majority of government benefits of all kinds, including defense and homeland security, are financed largely by taxes levied on the working population.

Young people are not oblivious to the inequity at the root of our social safety net for older Americans. Some 70 percent of Generation X'ers believe that Social Security will not be available to help them fund their own retirement. More young Americans believe in UFOs than believe that Social Security and Medicare will be available to help them when they retire.[31]

Young people already face a widening gap between publicly guaranteed benefits and those provided by private firms. As unionization has receded, so has pressure from employers to provide health and retirement coverage for their workers. The plentiful supply of young workers provided by the baby boom made competition for new workers less urgent. As a consequence, increasing numbers of younger Americans (the nonelderly, nonpoor) lack both health insurance coverage and private pensions. Some 47 million Americans lacked health insurance at some time during 2006.[32] The largest percentage of uninsured in any age group comprises people between ages 18 and 24. Almost 59 percent of uninsured people worked full or part time and support, through their payroll tax deductions, today's older population regardless of their elders' economic need.[33]

The result of our legacy social programs and a thirty-year-long buyers' market for workers is a richly entitled older population, most of whom are no longer poor. As we will see, many are asset rich, both in real estate and in equities; yet their public benefits are subsidized by a younger population facing higher taxes, higher costs of living, and an ever-skimpier social safety net. How we reconfigure these subsidy flows to protect the smaller but still significant population of older Americans who remain economically vulnerable is the heart of the policy challenge.

Why the Catastropharians Are Wrong

What's wrong with the catastropharian scenario? First, the notion of a dependency ratio based on the relative size of "old" versus "young" age cohorts is a questionable construct. The term "dependency ratio" implies that those over age 65 are simply idle consumers of tax revenues supplied by younger workers. This is a bogus assumption.

People over age 50 own 70 percent of all financial assets in the country (well in excess of $10 trillion), and therefore pay most of the capital gains taxes on appreciation of those assets.[34] Those assets are, it is worth remembering, the growth capital for the U.S. economy. Much of the political debate about tax policy in the past two decades has been, at its core, a debate over how to encourage the productive deployment of that capital.

As a group, baby boomers are wealthy, but that wealth is not evenly distributed across the generation. The average household net worth of the early baby boomers (born between 1946 and 1953) was estimated at $390,000 in a 2006 paper prepared for the Social Security Administration.[35] The average wealth of the top quartile of the income distribution of the early boomers, the sector to which Robert Smallwood from the prologue belongs, is $940,000.

This study found that wealth is disproportionately concentrated in that subset of baby boomers who own their own businesses. There is also a steep education gradient in household wealth. The mean wealth of college graduates is almost four times that of a high school graduate, and the mean wealth of those with postgraduate degrees is almost eight times that of those who did not finish high school.

The boomers in that top quartile are not merely going to sit on their wealth, clipping coupons or reinvesting their dividends, and then liquidating them when they cross the magic threshold of age 65. In part because much wealth is concentrated in the top quartile of the generation, boomers will probably not have to liquidate their wealth to pay their living expenses; rather, they will continue using it to capitalize much of our nation's future economic growth.[36] They will also spend rather than save their current income. Tomorrow's aging boomers will play a major role in generating jobs for younger workers. This relationship is symbiotic, not parasitic.

Nor do all intergenerational income transfers flow from the young to the old. A recent essay by Charles Mann suggested that public revenue transfers from younger to older Americans through Social Security and Medicare may have been offset by hidden but substantial direct revenue flows from parents to young people *within* families.[37]

These revenue flows have been increasing in recent years as housing costs rise, wages in the service sector stagnate, and adolescence lengthens into the 30s. The parents of perpetual adolescents are transferring wealth inside their families to support their children's living costs, at the cost of their children's autonomy. Twenty-five percent of adults between the ages of 18 and 34 now live with their parents, according to the 2000 U.S. census. An estimated 18 million young adults are out of college but not living on their own.[38]

Second, past is not prologue. Boomers have very different plans for their lives from their parents and grandparents. The major difference between baby boomers and their elders is that most boomers expect to continue working long past age 65—many part time, but a surprising number, about 7 percent, full time.[39] Some 15 percent expect to start new businesses after they "retire" from their current job. These work plans will be supported by improved health status of older people, permitting longer working careers.

Through the taxes they pay both on the income generated by the trillions in assets they own and on their working wages after age 65, baby boomers will be helping to fund a larger-than-anticipated share of their own social and private benefits, as well as paying for the less fortunate members of their own generation. Much of the presumed intergenerational burden decried by the catastropharians may well be financed by *intra*generational income transfers inside the baby boom itself for *decades*. The magnitude and implications of this "new" older work force is discussed at length in the next chapter.

Nor does the "dependency ratio" account for the significant noneconomic effort of older Americans—from volunteering to unpaid caregiving. Rowe and Kahn estimated that 40 percent of people 55 or older reported more than 1,500 hours a year of "productive activity" (which includes volunteer work) and another 40 percent spent between 500 and 1,500 hours.[40] The idea of classifying people over a certain age as "dependent" on the younger population merely because of their age is both offensive and misleading. Many younger boomers will be caring for their older boomer spouses, relatives, and others in the community, as well as helping less-fortunate younger people through volunteer efforts.

Third, though there is a large demographic pause following the baby boom, the decline in the number of people born after 1964 reversed itself in the 1980s (see figure 1.1). The rebound in the U.S. birthrate produced a substantial baby boom "echo," which began in 1977.[41] The echo boom is much larger than the baby boom, though it is spread over a longer time span—108 million versus 76 million for the original baby boom. The thirteen years after 1964 created a demographic "valley" between the baby boom and the echo boom. Crossing this valley will be a labor market and fiscal challenge, but it is not necessarily a threshold to a permanently older society (as we will see in much of Europe). The extent to which this is so will depend on both immigration trends and the length of the echo boom.

As echo boomers enter the labor market, their earning power and tax revenues generated by their economic activity will be available to subsidize the costs of the fragile subset of the baby boom (to which Avril Sanchez from our prologue belongs) and eventually the older boomers' final years. When echo boomers move into their prime earning years, the fiscal capacity of the country to absorb the health and income security costs of the baby boom will increase significantly.

Immigration rates also affect the tax base. Population estimates for the year 2000 were some 5 million lower than the actual 2000 census results, in large measure because of the underestimated rate of immigration into the United States and the higher birthrates of migrants versus legacy residents. In addition to legal immigrants, who are easy to count, there are an estimated 12 million immigrants in the country illegally, most of them employed or seeking work.[42] Interestingly, owing to this growth in immigration and the echo boom, the proportion of people over age 65 actually *fell* in the United States from 1990 to 2005 (from 12.5% to 12.4%).[43]

The United States has for its entire history been a beacon for ambitious people from all over the world. Tens of millions of people in other countries that lack the economic and political freedoms of the United States continue to view our country as the land of opportunity. Despite the challenges posed by global terrorism, ours remains an open economy and society. A major opportunity for alleviating looming shortages of workers in the U.S. labor market is to admit more foreign workers. Notwithstanding present anxieties about immigrants stealing jobs from current American workers, shortages of skilled and unskilled labor in the United States will eventually overwhelm the current political opposition to immigration.

This Isn't Your Grandfather's Economy

As we look forward twenty years, it is important to recognize how different the challenge we face in the next thirty years is from the scary near-death social and economic experience of the 1930s. Reconstruction of a shattered economic base is not the main challenge for twenty-first-century American society. Rather, the United States is an economic powerhouse, albeit one in need of a higher savings rate and a renovated international image. Though its centrality is threatened by accumulating foreign debt and trade imbalances, the dollar remains the reserve currency of the world. The last serious countrywide recession in the United States was twenty-seven years ago.

The affordability of our safety net for older Americans turns on the prospects for future economic growth as well as the timing of the eventual costs of the baby boom's final act. A prosperous, growing country of 400 million people, a population that the United States is projected to reach by 2043,[44] will have a much more robust capacity to fund social programs for vulnerable seniors than a stagnant, struggling country of 320 million people. Measures that promote economic growth have as much saliency in funding our social safety net as managing the cost of our social promises.

One core element of the catastropharian argument is valid: the New Deal–Great Society programs are long overdue for renovation. Medicare, in particular, is broken, and its costs, indeed, its very rationale, need to be reframed, years before the first baby boomer enrolls. Fixing Medicare, in particular, is not a demographic imperative; unchecked health spending is today, not tomorrow, a threat to not only the federal budget but also the value of our currency.

No reasonable person wants to abolish the New Deal and Great Society programs; the security they provide is an indispensable foundation for a modern economy and compassionate society. Where

I part company with the catastropharians is in believing that the forthcoming generation of seniors differs fundamentally from those who have gone before them and that those differences matter profoundly in framing social policy. The assumptions we make about the future of the baby boomers—both their capabilities and their plans— ought to shape the prescription for renovating these important social programs.

The baby boom generation will be the most prosperous and best-educated group of older Americans since the founding of the Republic. The prosperous and highly educated seniors of tomorrow are going to be as different from those frightened Dust Bowl farmers fighting off the sheriff as Lauren Hutton and her motorcycle are from Granny Clampett and her shotgun.

In the next chapter, we consider the changing nature of work and why the concept of retirement has a fundamentally different saliency in a knowledge economy than in the manufacturing economy it replaced. To understand why I believe the catastropharians have it wrong, we need to understand better how baby boomers' life paths are likely to differ from those of their parents and grandparents. Once this is better understood, we can construct a more likely societal scenario than the presumed "mass retirement at age 65" that drives much of the catastropharian nightmare and then discuss its policy ramifications.

three

Living to Work

Boomers, Retirement, and the Knowledge Economy

Although key social programs in the United States have not changed materially in the decades since they were enacted, the U.S. economy of 2006 is far different. The agrarian-industrial economy of the 1930s and the manufacturing economy of the years following World War II have given way to a knowledge economy, employing a work force far more educated than any in this (or any other) country's history.

That knowledge economy grew out of postwar America's love affair with higher education. Baby boomers' parents established the pathway to advanced education upon returning from the war through participation in the GI Bill. After its enactment by Congress in 1944, the GI Bill provided $14.5 billion in support for World War II veterans seeking higher education and another $4.5 billion for Korean War veterans.[1] More than 10 million baby boomer parents gained access to higher education as a result. Many boomer parents passed on to their children a legacy of expectations that they, too, would not only finish college but even seek an advanced degree.

Investment in higher education, as well as in research and development, received a further powerful boost from geopolitical competition with the Soviet Union. The USSR shocked the United States in 1957 by launching a tiny satellite called Sputnik into Earth orbit.

Sputnik symbolized the advance of Soviet science and technology into the threshold of space and came at a time of high anxiety over the arms race between the United States and the Soviet Union. Rallying against this perceived military threat, the United States aggressively invested in scientific research and training, as well as launched the space program. President Kennedy committed to putting a man on the moon by the end of the 1960s. This commitment was supported by increased funding for the National Science Foundation, the founding of the Defense Advanced Research Projects Agency (DARPA), and aggressive expansion of training grants for science education to expand the cadre of Ph.D.-level scientists.

The results were stunning: a doubling in higher educational enrollments from 1965 to 1975. Approximately 500 new colleges and university campuses were created during this period.[2] This enrollment increase, in turn, created approximately 140,000 new jobs in the higher educational sector, including a rapidly expanding community college system, to accommodate the new student demand.

Enrollments in higher education were further swollen by military draft policies during the Vietnam conflict. For most of the 1960s, the Selective Service System gave deferments for male students pursuing a college or graduate degree. Many young men anxious to avoid being sent to Vietnam stayed in college or graduate school to shelter themselves from conscription. These deferments were eliminated in 1971, when this system, which discriminated against the poor and those from working-class backgrounds, was replaced by a universal draft lottery.

Graduate scientific and technical education lengthened the higher educational experience and swelled the flow of highly trained scientific and technical workers into the U.S. economy. The number of workers with master's degrees expanded by 142 percent and with academic doctoral degrees by 106 percent from 1965 to 1975.[3] This flood of highly trained workers became the shock troops for a new, knowledge-based economy.

Higher education served during the late 1960s and 1970s as a "flood-control reservoir" that gave the labor market some much-needed time to adjust to the flood of new young workers. The surge in higher education enrollments had the effect of first deferring the

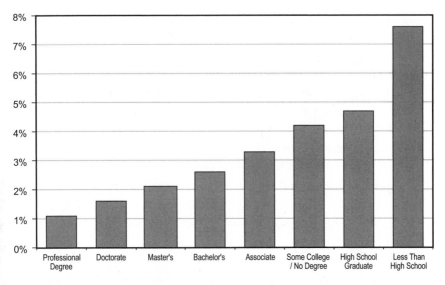

Figure 3.1. Unemployment rate, 2005
Source: Data from Bureau of Labor Statistics.

baby boom's entry into the work force and then releasing millions of workers whose college or advanced degree attainments overqualified them for a limited amount of skilled positions.

As the economy struggled in the 1970s and 1980s to absorb tens of millions of new workers, the baccalaureate degree and advance degrees became gateways to many jobs that did not strictly require advanced training. The unemployment rate for people with college and advanced degrees, while very low compared to that of high school dropouts, reached historic levels during the 1970s, giving rise to concerns about whether the U.S. economy was making effective use of its highly trained work force. By 2005, however, the higher one's level of educational attainment, the lower the risk of unemployment (figure 3.1).

Worker Mobility

The nature of employment changed dramatically during this period as well. The early twentieth-century idea that a person worked for a single large firm for his or her entire life gave way to increasing worker mobility among firms. As the economy grew in the 1980s, a no-madic career path replaced the "single firm–company town" paradigm that drove the industrial economy. Economic power shifted from the company to the knowledge worker, and from the large to the small firm. Almost three-quarters of the job growth from 1990 to 1995 came not from Fortune 500 firms but from firms of fewer than 500 employees.[4]

Both occupational and physical mobility are deeply ingrained in the baby boomer life-style. U.S. workers today change jobs every five to seven years. The younger the worker, the more the mobility.[5] Every year, more than 24 million Americans change jobs. Approximately 40 million Americans move *every year,* in pursuit of a new job or for other reasons.[6] This type of mobility—both between jobs and be-tween communities—is one important way the U.S. economy differs from those in Europe.

With the election of Ronald Reagan and elevation of entrepreneur-ship to a civic virtue, starting a business became a socially valued al-ternative to working for someone else. Millions of new firms were created during the past twenty years of the twentieth century, as busi-ness ownership replaced employment as the career goal of many baby boomers.

Baby Boom Women: Storming the Labor Market

An important change that attended the baby boom's entrance into the labor market was a marked increase in the labor force participa-tion rate of women. This mass entrance was linked to the broad avail-ability of reliable contraception, as well as access to legal abortion after *Roe v. Wade* in 1973. Oral contraceptives introduced in the 1960s made having a family truly optional and gave boomer women an explicit choice their mothers and grandmothers did not have. About 14 percent of the women married between 1880 and 1910 did not have children. By 1930, only 7 percent of married women did not have children.

This trend reversed for baby boomers, as 24 percent of women married in the 1960s and 1970s did not have children.[7] The age at first marriage also increased dramatically, to 25 for those born in

1957.[8] And family size, as well as the amount of time women needed to spend on child rearing, fell significantly as boomer women exercised their new choices.

The drop in family size, the large number of boomer women electing not to have children, and the rise in female labor force participation rates are inextricably linked. Baby boom women showed sharply higher labor force participation rates than their mothers and grandmothers. Fifty percent of women born between 1926 and 1935 (boomer parents) were in the labor force by midlife. This jumped to nearly 77 percent for early baby boomer women (figure 3.2).[9] This much-higher labor force participation by women meant a far higher "full-time equivalent" impact of the baby boom on the U.S. work force than that produced by population growth alone.

The cumulative effect of these changes was to move work to virtually equal footing with family in the boomer hierarchy of values. As the birthrate fell and increasing numbers of boomer families either postponed having children or had one child—in contrast to their par-

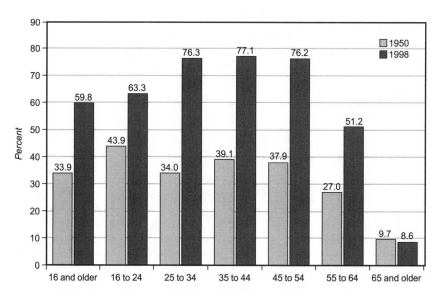

Figure 3.2. Labor force participation rates of women, by age, 1950 and 1998
Source: H. N. Fullerton Jr., "Labor Force Participation: 75 Years of Change, 1950–98 and 1998–2025," Monthly Labor Review, December 1999, pp. 3–12.

ents, who may have had three or more—baby boomers reallocated their time and energy to their jobs.

The Centrality of Work to Boomers' Lives

Today, the average American worker works more than 1,800 hours a year, compared to about 1,500 hours for the average European (figure 3.3). Part of this difference is accounted for by labor laws in European countries that mandate generous vacation and sick leave for all employees, as well as limit the duration of the workweek. American workers are also among the most productive in the world, and that productivity gap appears to be widening.

Important cultural differences with other societies undergird the higher level of commitment Americans have to work. More than family, class, clan, religion, language or community, what Americans do for a living confirms their social identity. In defining who someone is, work plays a more central role in the contemporary United States than perhaps anywhere else in the world.

Work became a vital conduit of not only wealth but also prestige and social meaning in the boomer-dominated late twentieth-century

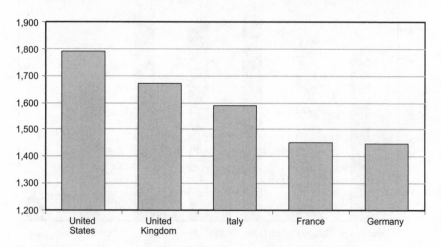

Figure 3.3. Annual hours worked per person in employment
Source: OECD Employment Outlook, 2004. www.oecd.org/document/62/0,2340,
en_2649_201185_31935102_1_1_1_1,00.html.

U.S. economy. Work provides not only meaning to most boomers' lives but also the network of social relationships that is central to their lives. In the United States, workaholics are venerated rather than pitied. As David Brooks put it in *Bobos in Paradise,* "In the 1960s, most social theorists assumed that as we got richer, we would work less and less. But if work is a form of self-expression or a social mission, then you never want to stop"[10] (see figure 3.4).

This is not meant to imply that all baby boomers love their jobs. A Conference Board survey in 2005 suggested that a little less than half of workers aged 45–54 are satisfied with their jobs. Job satisfaction is strongly correlated with both age and salary, suggesting that, over time, people tend to migrate to jobs that gratify them. Yet approximately one-quarter of the U.S. work force is "simply showing up to collect a paycheck."[11]

This centrality of work in boomers' lives becomes crucial because the presumed mass withdrawal of baby boomers from the labor

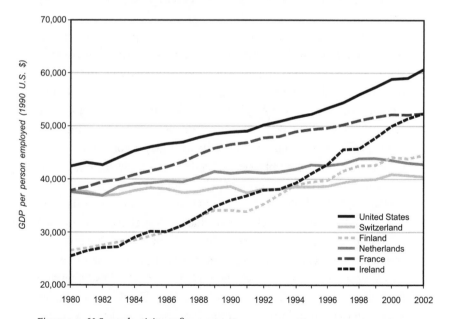

Figure 3.4. U.S. productivity, 1980–2002
Source: *Adapted from Key Indicators of the Labour Market,* 5th ed. (Geneva: International Labour Office, 2007).

market and their consequent dependence on society for their support play a central role in the catastropharian scenario. Whereas some boomers do look forward to retirement, many more seem likely to be completely lost if they are not working at something. Many baby boom workers who are dissatisfied with their present jobs will view "retirement" not as a time to cease working but rather as a time to find work (paid or unpaid) that better fits their values and dreams.

The Golden Years: A Post–World War II Idea

The concept of the "golden years," a period of leisure at the end of life comparable to an extended, dry-land version of a ship cruise, is a mid-twentieth-century idea. It was wedded to a labor market dominated by physically demanding and mentally unchallenging manufacturing employment. In the *pre*industrial labor market of primarily commercial and agricultural employment, workers (who were either self-employed or very-low-wage employees) simply worked until they dropped.

The idea of retirement became popular during the postwar economic boom, when the growth in manufacturing employment substantially strengthened the role of unions in guaranteeing worker benefits, including pensions. As late as 1950, 34 percent of all jobs were in manufacturing.[12] At one point in the early 1950s, a little more than a third of U.S. workers were members of labor unions, compared to 12 percent in 2006 (and many of the latter-day union members are actually government employees). Of today's private-sector U.S. workers, only 7.4 percent are represented by labor unions.[13]

Through the collective-bargaining process, labor unions won guaranteed pensions, which, when added to Social Security, enabled large numbers of workers to retire at age 65 or earlier. The ability of unions to confer health and retirement benefits for their members was almost more important symbolically than their ability to bargain for higher wages. Workers could point to these benefits as a tangible return on their contribution of union dues. As late as the early 1950s, some 46 percent of men older than 65 were in the labor market. During this next forty years, this number dropped to 17 percent.[14]

The economic cost of these retirement guarantees has today reached the point of threatening the survival of many of these companies, who are, in turn, offloading the burden onto taxpayers through the federal Pension Guarantee Board. According to a recent study by the U.S. comptroller general, more than 1,100 corporate pension plans are nearly $354 billion short of the funding they have promised to their workers, as of mid-2005.[15] As companies have been unable to fund the cost of these promises, federal guarantees of those pensions has spiraled to more than $21 billion.

Retiree health coverage is also in retreat, as the number of workers covered by retiree health programs fell dramatically, from 66 percent in 1988 to 36 percent in 2004.[16] This steep decline followed a 1990 decision by the Federal Accounting Standards Board requiring firms to reflect the future costs of their retiree benefits as liabilities on their balance sheets. After the steep plunge following the FASB decision, the percentage of firms offering retiree health coverage was actually dead flat from 1993 to 2004 at 36 percent. These large gaps in retiree income and health benefits will complicate the ability of many baby boomers who might otherwise wish to retire before they are eligible for Medicare to do so.

As a social experiment, retirement does not appear have been an unalloyed success. Today's retirees—the parents and grandparents of baby boomers—watch a mind-numbing forty-three hours of television a week. One-half of today's retirees would rather be working, and one-third of those who retire in their 50s return to work within a few years, citing boredom and lack of fulfillment as a major reason.[17] Watching and living with their parents' retirement experiences is likely to have a catalytic effect on baby boomers' own plans for the last third of their lives.

The health status of the newly retired is well known to deteriorate sharply at the point of retirement, and not merely because some people retire for health reasons. Idleness after a lifetime of work coincides with the onset of depression, weight gain, marital tension, and a variety of other stressful conditions. Mortality risk increases sharply in the immediate postretirement years.[18] The suicide rate among those newly retired also spikes sharply. Overall, the suicide rate among older Americans is higher than that of their children; whereas those older than 65 constitute only 13 percent of all Americans, they account for almost 20 percent of all suicides.[19]

Over 65: A Diverse Population

The population over 65 today, baby boomers' parents and their younger siblings, is far from homogeneous. In a survey of retirees conducted with Harris Interactive in 2002, gerontologist Ken Dychtwald divided the present retiree population into four groups.[20] "Ageless Explorers," a subgroup he believes presages the boomers, constitutes 27 percent of the population. These people with active life-styles have continued working and simply do not identify themselves as "old." Another group, about 19 percent of the survey sample, termed "Comfortably Content," represents people who have settled into the Golden Years vision of retirement and are enjoying a life of leisure. A third group, roughly 22 percent, that Dychtwald termed "Live for Todays," comprises those who lead fun, interesting lives, but have not made adequate provision for retirement and have uncertain futures because they lack the resource base to continue living at their present standard indefinitely.

Finally, Dychtwald found a large group of older Americans, about *one-third* of his sample, whom he terms "Sick and Tireds" and characterizes as "beaten down by life and having a miserable time in retirement." They have limited financial resources and health problems and are basically running out the clock and, I strongly suspect, making those around them miserable while they do it.

The centrality of work in the lives of baby boomers will fundamentally alter their life plans. It is highly unlikely that baby boomers will follow their parents out to pasture. Most baby boomers have different attitudes toward retirement than their parents do. In two surveys of baby boomer attitudes toward retirement, AARP found a small group, perhaps 13 percent of boomers they termed "enthusiasts," people who cannot wait to retire and do not plan on working after they retire. AARP also identified a larger group of boomers called "traditionalists," perhaps 20 percent of boomers; who plan on working (mostly part time) but are nonetheless confident in the solidity of the safety net programs.

Only 16 percent of baby boomers surveyed in 2002, however, said they planned on not working after age 65; the remaining 84 percent said that they would work after 65, "even if they were set for life."[21] How much of this will be making a virtue of a necessity remains to be seen, as many boomers are underreserved, overleveraged, and not thinking seriously about twenty years from now. Those among today's workers who expect to work after retirement because they want to outnumber those who expect to work because they have to; of workers aged 50 or older, 52 percent are in the former group, and 30 percent in the latter.[22]

Both groups—the traditional retirement aficionados and those who expect to work at least part time—believe that Social Security and Medicare will be there to support them and will be key to maintaining their living standards. They have some private retirement funding and savings, and their needs are relatively modest. I refer to this large middle group, about one-third of the baby boom, as "Might Be OK" baby boomers—as in "Might be OK if they make the right financial and health-related choices." (Peter Porter, from the prologue, is a "Might Be OK" baby boomer.)

There are two other important groups of boomers. The most worrisome are those who not only are inadequately provisioned to retire but also may be unable to continue working into their 60s or 70s, regardless of their wishes. Approximately one-third of boomers fall into this category. They lack savings because they spend their entire current incomes (and then some) on living expenses and coping with health and other problems. Many of them have experienced the wealth-destroying events of divorce and illness or disability long before they attained traditional retirement age. They lack sufficient retirement savings and home equity to function without Social Security and Medicare. Many of them are barely getting by today, sinking deeper into personal debt.

The lower-income part of this group AARP terms "strugglers," about 15 percent of the total boomer population. They have much lower family income than any other group. Though the AARP surveys did not probe specifically for health status, many members of this group likely struggle with alcoholism, depression, and physical disabilities such as obesity or lower back problems and may be unable to continue working long into their 60s even if they wish to do so. Almost 16 percent of today's 45- to 64-year-olds already have a limitation in usual activities. More than 13 percent, approximately 9.4 million, of those aged 45–54 are unable to work or are limited in their capacity to do so, which is about three times that of those aged 18–44 years.[23]

At the same time, the gap between what they spend and what Social Security, their sole income support for later in their lives, will cover is large enough that many will have to continue working. If they lose their jobs, their exclusive dependence on Social Security benefits will probably result in a sharp decline in their living standards, and perhaps their access to health care, and may push them into the sheltering arms of their adult children, if they have any.

Another troubled baby boomer cohort, whom AARP terms the "anxious," are better off than the "strugglers" and have been saving for retirement, but the combination of what they have put aside and what they will receive from Social Security and Medicare will probably not be adequate to meet their medical expenses (i.e. the portion presently not covered by Medicare). The "anxious" represent about 17 percent of the boomer population. Most of those in both groups expect to have to work past normal "retirement" age, even if they do not wish to work. Whether they are *able* to do so may be determined in major part by their health status and their skills and work experience. These two groups, which I call "Struggling and Anxious," pose the most significant public policy challenge within the baby boom population. (Avril Sanchez, from the prologue, is a "Struggling and Anxious" baby boomer.)

Finally, there is the fortunate one-third of boomers whose work plans and asset positions make at least Social Security largely irrelevant. AARP refers to this group as the "self-reliants." They have median family incomes of $82,000, more than 20 percent higher than the average for the boomers. Only 26 percent of this group would alter retirement or work plans if Medicare or Social Security were not available. I refer to this group as "Set for Life." This is meant not merely in an economic sense but in the sense that their health and energy will enable them to live a vigorous and active later life. This group includes the opinion leaders and shapers, political leaders, and knowledge worker elite not just of the baby boom generation but also of the whole society. They will likely serve as the public face of the baby boomers, even though they are a numerical minority in their generation. They are highly prominent in advertisements in AARP's flagship publication, *AARP, the Magazine*. (Richard Smallwood, from the prologue, is a "Set for Life" baby boomer.)

Because they lack pension coverage or the asset base to retire without suffering a sharp decline in their living standards, many baby boomers will have to continue working. Although only about 7 percent of boomer households have a present zero or negative household net worth, many other boomers have limited financial assets that will be threatened by unanticipated health care costs until they reach the age of eligibility for Medicare (and after). Indeed, the single greatest barrier to retirement *before* age 65 will be access to affordable health care coverage. Among workers over age 45, 65 percent said that maintaining health care coverage was a reason why they would continue working.[24] This issue will be a major focus of the needed policy changes to support longer work careers, which affects both Medicare and tax policy.

Free Agency and the Growing Obsolescence of Retirement

For tens of millions of baby boomers, retiring will mean "rewiring" rather than ceasing to work. Only 7 percent of boomers surveyed by AARP in 2003 said that retirement meant to them "not working."[25] Ken Dychtwald has long argued that, rather than retiring, most boomers will have serial careers and continue working long past traditional retirement age.[26] Many will work part time, but a surprising number of others plan on using their wealth and resource position to start new enterprises or to work in nonprofit or community benefit jobs. According to a recent AARP poll, 16 percent of older people plan to work for themselves or start their own business.[27]

Today, 6.8 million people over age 50 are self-employed, about one in five workers in this age group.[28] One-third became self-employed after age 50, which suggests that it is a significant career transition mechanism for those leaving salaried employment. Of those self-employed workers who are married, 42 percent work with their spouse.

Given that baby boomers were pioneers of the free-agent economy, the number of older workers who work for themselves will head sharply higher, as today's self-employed boomers extend their free agency into their 60s and beyond. Male labor force participation after age 65, which fell sharply in the United States beginning in the 1950s, reversed course in the early 1990s, a full twenty years ahead of the baby boom. As of 2003, 33 percent of men aged 65–69 worked, and 12 percent of men over age 70. Among women, 23 percent over age 65 worked, and 6 percent over age 70.[29] These participation rates will eventually double or increase even more as boomers reach these ages.

Japan, a society that is aging faster than the United States, already has significantly higher rates of labor force participation among older workers. The International Labor Organization says 71 percent of Japanese men ages 60 to 64 work, mostly in postretirement jobs. That compares with 57 percent of American men and just 17 percent of French men in the same age group.[30]

Baby boomer wealth will create career options for boomers that their parents and grandparents did not have. According to a recent Urban Institute study, the average "early boomer" household is projected to have a net worth of $854,000 by age 67, some 42 percent higher than that of their parents (figure 3.5). Later boomers, defined as those born after 1957, are projected to have only slightly lower net worth.[31] These assets are concentrated in the top quartile of boomers, with some huge fortunes buried in these averages. (Bill Gates is in there somewhere, but Warren Buffett's wealth is buried in the average wealth of the current retiree population.)

This remarkable resource position reflects two important developments: the ongoing roughly $10 trillion transfer of wealth from inheritance from baby boomers' parents and the remarkable appreciation in the value of real estate that began in earnest in the 1980s and accel-

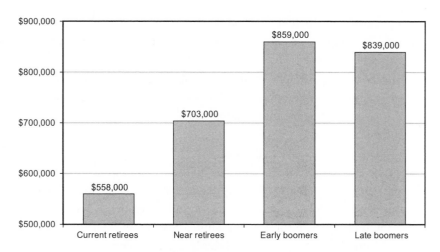

Figure 3.5. Average household wealth at age 67
Source: Urban Institute, Washington, D.C., May 2004.

erated in the wake of the tech stock market crash of 2001.[32] Much of
the inheritance wealth transfer will be in the form of real estate free of
mortgage, the value appreciation of which can be passed to children
free of taxation and then borrowed against. Real estate wealth is not
the sole source of baby boomer assets, however; there are also trillions
of dollars in equity in companies, both publicly and privately held.

This substantial base of wealth will create options for the millions
of boomer households, like Robert Smallwood's, fortunate enough to
have it. Though one option obviously includes a comfortable traditional retirement, boomer wealth also will help create new businesses
and nonprofit enterprises. For superwealthy boomers, in addition to
the opportunity to shelter capital gains from business investments,
tax incentives will encourage the creation of a new layer of charitable
foundations to support community benefit initiatives, which will employ not only fellow boomers but also their children.

The Coming Dearth of Skilled Workers

Even if baby boomers wished to cease working in large numbers,
the U.S. economy will not be able to afford to let them. Unlike the la-

bor markets of the mid-twentieth century, which were flooded with young workers, labor market conditions expected in the next twenty years will reinforce the baby boomer disposition to continue working. This is because, despite continuing substantial improvements in worker productivity, employers both public and private will not be able to replace retiring boomers one-for-one with experienced younger workers.

Thanks to the baby bust, a legacy of U.S. economic troubles during the 1970s, there is a gaping hole in the U.S. work force that will compromise the ability of many businesses, schools, health care providers, and other enterprises to continue operations. Beginning in the mid-1960s, fertility in the United States plummeted 50 percent, from the postwar peak of 3.8 children per couple to only 1.8 children per couple by 1975. By 2001, fertility rates had returned to 2.1 children born per couple, the same level as during the Great Depression. If boomers do retire at anything approximating the rate of their parents' generation, it will create an unprecedented human resource problem for a talent-hungry U.S. economy.[33]

The Bureau of Labor Statistics forecast that there will be 10 million more jobs than workers in the U.S. labor market by 2010 (some of which will be filled by people working two jobs) (figure 3.6). In February 2007 the unemployment rate for workers with college degrees was only 1.9 percent.[34] The market for skilled labor is already exceptionally tight and will grow far tighter as the next fifteen years unfold. By 2010 the leading edge of the baby boom will not yet have reached the traditional retirement age of 65. A National Association of Manufacturers survey projected a 5.3 million person shortage of *skilled* labor in 2010, but a 14 million shortage by 2020, when the youngest boomers are nearing or have reached age 60.[35]

Government employers may be the hardest hit. According to a recent General Accountability Office (GAO) analysis of federal work force needs, 60 percent of 1.6 million white-collar federal employees and 90 percent of the 6,000-person federal executive work force will be eligible to retire within ten years.[36] The average age of the federal employee increased from 42.3 years in 1990 to 46.5 in 2001. In

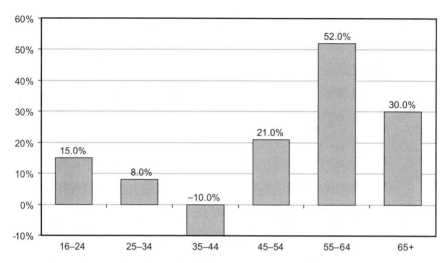

Figure 3.6. Growth in the U.S. work force by age group, 2000–2010
Source: Bureau of Labor Statistics, 2001.

2003, 22 percent of the federal work force was already at or above the minimum retirement age of 55, but only 6 percent was below the age of 30.[37]

Almost half of the air traffic controllers in the United States will reach *mandatory* retirement age by 2011. Although their mandatory retirement age is 56, federal law provides for exemptions, up to age 61, for controllers with exceptional skills and experience. The GAO predicts that about 600–800 controllers will leave each year between 2002 and 2011. It also indicates that about 37 percent of the current controller work force is projected to leave by 2011.[38]

State governments could lose more than 30 percent of their work force to retirement, private-sector employment, or alternative careers by 2006, and health agencies would be the hardest hit.[39] Currently, some 20 percent of elementary and secondary school teaching positions in the country are vacant, and in 2000 the average age of public school teachers was 42.[40] Recent surveys suggest that 40 percent of the current cadre of elementary and secondary school teachers expect not to be teaching in K–12 schools five years from now.[41]

The Health Care System's Need for Skilled Workers

The health care system provided millions of new jobs for the baby boom generation, and it continued expanding aggressively during the first decade of the twenty-first century. A recent *Business Week* survey (2006) suggested that the health care system was responsible for 1.7 million new jobs since the turn of the century, a figure that was equivalent to the number of net new private-sector jobs created by the U.S. economy at that time.[42]

The health care system's labor force crisis point is not projected to occur in a decade; it is already upon us. And it is not driven by rising boomer health care needs. Decades before the baby boomers reach the hospital in significant numbers as patients, baby boom–vintage hospital workers will have moved on to other, less-stressful employment.

Vacancy rates for nurses in the nation's hospitals reached the low teens in 2001, while the average age of RNs is 47 years.[43] Vacancy rates for pharmacists, radiology technicians, laboratory workers, and other vital technical personnel in hospitals reached the midteens as of 2001, though they fell somewhat in the wake of a mild recession. The situation is likely to worsen as hospitals are finding recruitment of these professionals increasingly difficult. In addition, costs for nursing recruitment and retention have increased.[44] Though enrollment in nursing schools is up about 15 percent since 2000, these increases are not nearly sufficient to cover the expected departure of boomer nurses.

The supply crisis is likely to be acute among physicians as well as nurses. Some 38 percent of today's practicing physicians are over 50, and recent surveys have suggested that owing to burnout and disillusionment with the present health insurance system, as many as one-third of these physicians plan on leaving practice within five years, well short of the career length of the prior generation of physicians.[45]

Some of the 24/7 medical specialties, such as general surgery, neurosurgery, and cardiology, have already reached the point where they are not generating replacement levels of new physicians, creating crises of access to care for the nation's emergency rooms.[46] The disciplines that are not filling their residency match requirements tend to be in life-style-compromising specialties, in which workloads are unpredictable and tend to impinge on family and leisure activities[47]

Before it disbanded, the Council on Graduate Medical Education declared an impending physician shortage and recommended the number of physicians entering residency training each year increase from approximately 24,000 in 2002 to 27,000 in 2015.[48] In 2005 the Association of American Medical Colleges, which represents the nation's medical schools and teaching hospitals, recommended increasing medical school enrollments by 15 percent over the next ten years to cope with an emerging crisis of access to physicians.[49]

The health care system's most serious long-term problem is that the baby boom cohort of caregivers will have found other employment just as an increasing number of older patients with chronic disease enter the system. Unless the health care system can manage fundamental improvements in worker productivity, labor shortages alone could dramatically increase the already sky-high cost of U.S. health care by the time the baby boom generation is fully in the throes of chronic illness.

Valuing Older Workers

The coming shortage of skilled workers is going to require a fundamental rethinking of employment policy toward older workers. Employers who wish to weather the coming shortage of workers will have to redesign work roles and rethink their present retirement policies, pension structure, and other barriers to continued employment of older workers. Present federal tax and pension policies contain significant barriers to work redesign and discourage employers from creating new work roles for older workers.

Eugene Steuerle, of the Urban Institute, said that "people in their late 50's, 60's and 70's have now become the largest underused pool of human resources in the economy."[50] According to Steuerle, the effect on the increasing labor force participation of older workers in the next twenty years will be as pronounced as that of women in the previous thirty years.

The free-agent economy, which baby boomers helped create, will enable large numbers of boomers to be self-employed and to be deployed in a flexible fashion to fill the gaps in the work force as long as their creativity and knowledge are in demand. It is unrealistic to expect that boomers will match perfectly with the skill needs of the emerging U.S. labor market, particularly in high-stress or physically demanding jobs. Boomer workers exiting these jobs in the next twenty years will create significant pressure on employers and labor markets. However, the flexible deployment of baby boomers' talents can help close some of the gaps in other areas, particularly government, education, and the professions.

Surviving the coming dearth of workers in the U.S. economy will also require rethinking Social Security and Medicare coverage policy, which continues, though not as dramatically as in the past, to contain disincentives for older Americans to continue working.

Immigration policy is also critical. In the catastropharian scenario, it is a wild card, because the alleged fiscal crisis of tomorrow is created in part by the 1970s fall in the U.S. domestic birthrates. During the tech boom of the 1990s, *legal* immigrants to the United States, particularly those from India and China, filled many of the skill positions in the U.S. workforce and created many of the new firms in information technology and services. Immigration rates for skilled workers, after rising sharply during the 1990s, contracted markedly in the spasm of xenophobia and bureaucratic complexity that followed 9/11. Whether this can be permitted to continue, given the global market for talent, is an urgent policy challenge.[51]

That boomers will follow their elders into retirement under the same ground rules as in the past forty years is the core flawed assumption of the catastropharian scenario. Boomers plan to continue working, and paying taxes, both longer and in far larger numbers than anticipated. Further, the wealth they have accumulated will be not passive wealth, but active wealth that creates jobs and opportunities for more of those younger workers. In the next chapter, I discuss what will enable longer and more productive work careers—namely, a steady improvement in the health status of older Americans.

four

Healthy Aging

Enabling a Longer, More Active Life

Contemporary images link aging with infirmity and dependence on others. A major determinant of the likely fate of the baby boom is how a longer life expectancy will affect the quality of baby boomers' lives as well as their ability to work and live independently at an advanced age. Here too, the catastropharians have gotten it wrong.

During the twentieth century, U.S. citizens added some thirty years to their average life expectancy compared to only ten years in the previous century. A woman born in 1900 could expect to live an average of forty-seven years; by the end of the twentieth century, she could expect to live seventy-eight years. This increase is the largest recorded in human life-span in a century in human history.[1]

The change occurred not merely in the United States; it happened across the modern world. We can actually trace the trend of increasing worldwide life expectancy, virtually in a straight line, back to 1840. Since that time, with remarkable constancy, we have added three months of average gain in life expectancy per year of elapsed time.[2] Given the chaos and brutality of the twentieth century, particularly the famines and epidemics that afflicted Africa, the two world wars, and totalitarian regimes in China and the Soviet Union that liquidated tens of millions of their citizens, it is extraordinary that the average life expectancy continued growing at all, let alone with such linear fixity.

If you are a catastropharian, however, this remarkable trend is bad news. Catastropharians associate aging with infirmity and disease, and a lengthened life-span with an increasing fiscal burden. Catastropharians have been influenced by the "failures of success" thesis of the gerontologist E. M. Gruenberg, propounded in 1977.[3] This gloomy theory of aging argues that we have purchased increased life expectancy at a terrible price: a lengthening period of illness and dependency at the end of life.

Those who subscribe to this theory believe that, by lengthening our life-span, we have increased the number of years in which we will be dependent on others—wearing diapers and being pushed around in wheelchairs by three shifts of caregivers, or warehoused in nursing homes. Because coping with this increased burden of disease through an expensive health care system will require spending a lot of money, increased life expectancy is seen as an inexorably growing fiscal burden to society.

The Improving Health of Older Americans

The real story of the emerging fate of the nation's older population is more complex, and the news is a good deal better: the health status of older Americans has improved significantly as their life-spans have lengthened. In other words, longer life-spans have meant longer periods of healthy life and reduced dependency on others, as well as a reduction in health expenses that would have occurred absent the improvements.

Most of the gain in life expectancy seen in the early twentieth century was the result of eliminating the premature causes of death—reducing infant mortality and controlling many of the infectious diseases (largely through public health measures) that killed people early in their lives. At the same time, there were, at best, modest increases in the *maximum* life-span.

There is strong circumstantial evidence that the maximum life-span may be determined in major part by genetic factors that limit the resiliency of our tissues and organ systems. The chronic diseases that claim most of us in old age are, first and foremost, dis-

eases that result from the declining ability of our organ systems—
degenerative diseases such as arthritis, osteoporosis, heart disease,
diabetes, Alzheimer's disease, and Parkinson's disease.

In 1980 James Fries of Stanford University posed an alternative to
Gruenberg's "failures of success" thesis. Fries argued that, rather
than experiencing declining health as we age, we would see improvement in the health status of older people. Because the maximum life-
span probably was not going to lengthen significantly, the result
would be a shortened period of morbidity at the end of life. If this
were true, rather than a lengthy compromised twilight, older people
would live a longer "functional" life and then die relatively quickly. In
Fries's view, older people would experience expanded life chances
and greater resiliency at the end of life.[4]

It appears that Fries was right and the doomsayers were wrong. By
analyzing long-term trend data on health status among older Americans, Duke University's Kenneth Manton established that disability
rates of older people declined at an accelerating rate from 1982 to
2004–5. Declines in disability averaged a little more than 1 percent
per year in the late 1980s, doubling to 2.2 percent per year in the last
five-year period.[5]

According to Manton's analysis, declines in disability were most
significant for the oldest age group. The proportion of those older
than 85 with no disability rose by almost one-third, to *more than half*
of the population, while the proportion of the oldest old who were institutionalized fell by a remarkable 43 percent. In the likelihood that
these declines continue for five more years at the average rate of the
past twenty years, 2009 Medicare spending will be $73 billion lower
than if the 1982 disability rates had been unchanged.[6] These data do
not, of course, yet include a single baby boomer.

Fries and other researchers have tied these gains in health status
to steady increases in the educational level of older people over the
past several decades.[7] According to Fries, lifetime cumulative disability was 20–60 percent lower for those over age 50 with higher education levels compared to age peers of lower educational attainment.
The effect of educational level was most pronounced, for both sexes,

over age 80, but particularly for males. Higher educational levels are associated with better health habits, more vigilance about early signs of preventable illness, and greater compliance with therapeutic guidelines and advice by physicians.[8]

This relationship will have particular saliency for baby boomers, who, as was previously discussed, have far higher levels of educational attainment than their parents or grandparents. If Manton's trend of declining disability rates remains intact for another twenty years, the younger boomers who reach 65 in 2030 may well be considered biologically to be "late middle age" rather than "elderly." Rather than being dependent on others, millions more boomers will be able to lead fulfilling and independent lives well into their 80s.

Can Technology Add to Our Functional Life-Span?

As this book is being written, the medical care system is in the process of building a new tool set to accelerate the improvements in functional life-span that Manton identified. Over the next few decades, clinicians will acquire the capacity to repair previously irreversible declines in functioning of key organ systems, the hallmark of the aging process. This emerging capability in medicine is called "regenerative medicine." The area of greatest progress has been in orthopedics and reconstructive surgery, in which replacement tissues for repair of burns, ligaments and tendons, bones, and facial features such as noses and ears are becoming available for surgical implantation.[9] Repair of herniated disks, damaged knee and shoulder ligaments and bones, and accelerated healing from broken bones will also grow rapidly in the next decade.[10] These latter developments will be of particular importance, given the ubiquity of arthritis among older people, as well as the threats posed by falls and broken hips.

Scientists are working intensively on the more difficult tasks of developing replacement tissues for the spinal cord, brain, and other nervous system structures that are damaged by trauma, stroke, and degenerative neurological illnesses such as Parkinson's disease and Alzheimer's disease. The ability to repair damage to the human heart by myocardial infarction (heart attack) and congestive heart failure (ischemic heart disease) is also under rapid and intensive development.[11] Damage to the heart and brain are two currently irrevocable losses that constitute major limiting factors on the lives of older people.

Research progress in understanding the molecular mechanisms of cell and tissue growth is vital to the development of regenerative medicine. If that progress continues apace, regenerative medicine may well develop sufficiently in the remaining lifetimes of younger boomers to affect their functional life-spans. Scientific advances in cell culture and cell therapy will dramatically broaden the scope of elective orthopedic care beyond the current practices in sports medicine, as well as expand reconstructive surgery, both of which have already expanded explosively in the past twenty years.[12] If the past two decades of Manton's trend may have been attributed to higher educational levels in the population and improved management of chronic illnesses, future improvements in functional life-span may be augmented by new science adapted and used by the medical care system.

Moreover, progress in the management of the major chronic illnesses that affect older Americans has resulted in marked reductions in death rates of two of the major killers of Americans—heart disease and stroke—and a gradual but accelerating reduction in the death rate from cancer, the most intractable of these illnesses (figure 4.1). The significant long-term reductions in death rates from heart disease appear to have been the result of improved clinical management of the disease.[13] However, recent declines in heart attack admissions to hospitals[14] suggest that widespread adoption of statin drugs and antihypertensive medications may be affecting the prevalence of the disease.

We may be surprised at the large numbers of baby boomers who survive to age 100 and beyond. Far from being basket cases, some of them could be still working.[15] The Census Bureau's 1999 estimates of approximately 850,000 centenarians were not its most aggressive

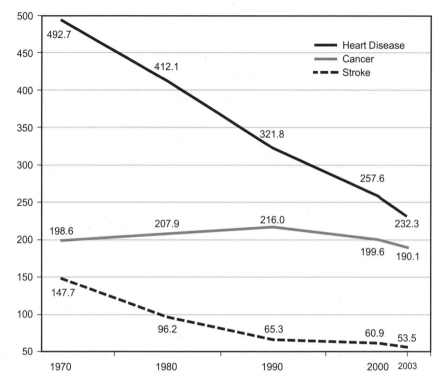

Figure 4.1. Leading causes of death for all ages, United States, 1970–2003 (deaths per 100,000)
Source: Centers for Disease Control and Prevention, National Center for Health Statistics, National Vital Statistics System.

forecasts; the high-end forecast was 4.2 million (figure 4.2).[16] These forecasts did not take into account much of the emerging technological progress in regenerative medicine and in scientific understanding of the molecular biology of aging.

These projections leave us in a very different place from the catastropharian vision. If the future forecast by these studies is borne out, improved health status will mean that tens of millions of baby boomers will be able to work and play and contribute far longer than their parents or grandparents. It will also mean continued reductions of in-hospital and nursing home use. Hospital use fell precipitously

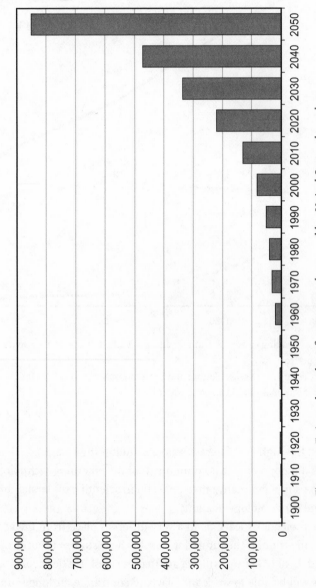

Figure 4.2. Estimated number of persons aged 100 or older, United States, through 2050

Source: U.S. Bureau of the Census, 1999.

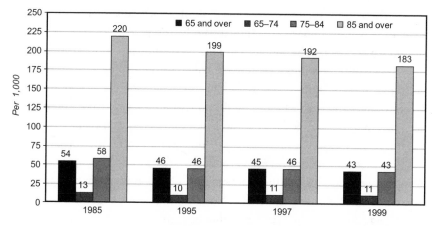

Figure 4.3. Rate of nursing home residence among people age 65 or older, by age group, 1985, 1995, 1997, and 1999

Note: Beginning in 1997, population figures are adjusted for net underenumeration using the 1990 National Population Adjustment Matrix from the U.S. Census Bureau. People residing in personal care or domiciliary care homes are excluded from the numerator. These data refer to the resident population.

Source: Centers for Disease Control and Prevention, National Center for Health Statistics, National Nursing Home Survey.

for older Americans in the past twenty years.[17] Nursing home use, per Manton, also fell (figure 4.3).

How Can Improving the Health Status for Older People Be Bad News?

How can this possibly be bad news for our society? Well, if you work at it, you can find the "crisis." Charles Mann, in a recent catastropharian treatise in the *Atlantic Monthly* entitled "The Coming Death Shortage," suggested that unequal access to life-extending medical care will place tremendous pressure on the Medicare program to make coverage of much of "regenerative medicine" universal.[18] Mann also suggests that older people who stay healthier longer will rob younger workers of economic opportunities by staying in their jobs longer.

There are numerous problems with Mann's zero-sum argument. One has already been mentioned: the looming critical shortage of skilled workers. Baby boomers will not be stealing jobs from younger workers if there will not be enough skilled workers to meet the economy's needs. The revealed preference of baby boomers to continue working, rather than becoming dependent on their children and on government subsidies, is a social blessing, not a curse. If the economy continues expanding as most forecasters expect, there will be great need for older workers to remain in the labor force longer, and not merely in jobs like the greeters at Wal-Mart. If the labor demand were shrinking or even static, Mann's argument about depriving young people of opportunities would have more validity.

Another problem with the argument is the strong likelihood that many older Americans will be able to use their own resources to pay for regenerative medicine, as many do today for cosmetic surgery or Lasik vision correction. The results will have fiscal consequences: they will be able to work longer and generate tax revenues that will help finance this type of care for the less-fortunate members of their own generation. On the other hand, many of these technologies may create sufficient social value that it makes sense for Medicare to pay for them.

A more recent and more thorough analysis of the cost impact of emerging technologies by Dana Goldman and colleagues at the Rand Corporation argued that, precisely *because* they will be effective in helping Americans live longer, *lifetime* Medicare spending will be increased. Goldman's study simulated the impact on Medicare spending of a variety of medical advances affecting chronic illness. The conclusion: "Some technologies are not expensive by themselves . . . , but add to health spending *because of their efficacy*. As people live longer, they incur more costs. Other technologies achieve health improvements at a very high price" (emphasis added).[19]

Given that Goldman's analysis seems to sweep away the societal benefits of potential innovations, such as a cure for cancer or a pill that halts the process of aging at the molecular level, and examines only their costs, this is a remarkable and unbalanced point of view. The real question is whether alleviating suffering and improving health status and outcomes for older people creates socioeconomic and personal value for them and their families that outweighs the cost of the innovation to society. These questions about new medical technologies we have been consistently unwilling to ask and answer rigorously. Rather, policy makers have tended in the past to assume that, if they are safe and effective, they must be worth whatever the innovator chooses to charge for them.[20] Then, policy makers and their colleagues in academia complain that, because the health care market basket is continuously expanding, society is not getting value received for the increased cost.

Many of the technologies, including some not considered in the Rand analysis, can significantly lower both the cost and the clinical risks of treating conditions affecting older people.[21] Leveraging these technologies to save money for Medicare will require changing Medicare's payment strategy to remove incentives to overtreat. Altering the incentives to health care providers, patients, and the technologies' developers to focus everyone more rigorously on producing social value would make Medicare a better social investment.

Even if technological advances are shown to add to lifetime Medicare expenses (because those who receive them live longer), postponing serious disability and illness is, as Martha Stewart would say, a good thing—not merely for boomers themselves but also, by reducing pressure on informal caregivers, for their spouses and children. It is also a macroeconomic victory, because it creates breathing room to allow the country's economy and fiscal capacity to grow. Postponing avoidable illness and health care costs is useful fiscally.

Goldman's model also may not accurately reflect the reality of what it costs to care for a healthier aged population. Lubitz and colleagues found that healthy people over age 70 not only live longer than their less-healthy age peers but actually generate less lifetime medical expenses, precisely because they use fewer health services. Lubitz concluded, "Health promotion efforts in the non-elderly population that have payoffs in better health and longer life for the elderly will not increase health spending among the elderly."[22] And the end-of-life costs for a person who lives to 90 years of age are about half of those for a person who dies young (in his late 60s).[23] This is a consequence of the "compression of morbidity" that Fries discussed: fragile older people die more quickly than younger people when challenged by disease. Far from being viewed as an economic risk, healthy aging should be pursued aggressively as a social policy objective.

Further, it is not the case that the only leverage to improve older Americans' health comes from expensive medical technology. Older Americans themselves can do a host of things to enhance the quality of their lives that cost the Medicare program nothing. There is a substantial and persuasive body of evidence that improved health habits, nutrition, and an active life-style could significantly increase the functional life-spans of older Americans. The most comprehensive review of this evidence is found in Rowe and Kahn's *Successful Aging*, which reports the results of a decade-long MacArthur Foundation study of what was known about the ability to improve the physical and mental abilities of older Americans.[24] Rowe and Kahn concluded that many conditions thought to be irrevocable functional losses due to aging could be not merely arrested but reversed by active management of disease risks and by encouraging more vigorous life-styles and social engagement of older Americans.

It follows directly that younger boomers who do not wait until their 60s to adopt health-improving diet, exercise, and medication patterns could do substantially better than their older boomer peers. These health changes will permit those younger boomers to stay on the job longer or to find new and more satisfying employment. The longer work lives will likely have the synergistic effect of keeping working boomers healthier longer.

What could interfere with these healthy developments? Two emerging health risks could conceivably deflect Manton's rising arc of health status among older Americans: obesity and Alzheimer's disease.

Will Obesity Spoil the Party?

Some gerontologists and health policy specialists recently raised a concern about whether the epidemic of obesity seen in the United States in the past twenty-five years will reverse Manton's trend and result in deteriorating health status among older people (table 4.1).

TABLE 4.1.

Increase in Prevalence of Overweight, Obesity, and Severe Obesity, as Measured by Body Mass Index, among U.S. Adults

	Overweight (BMI≥25)	Obesity (BMI≥30)	Severe Obesity (BMI≥40)
	(%)	(%)	(%)
1999–2000	64.5	30.5	4.7
1988–1994	56.0	23.0	2.9
1976–1980	46.0	14.4	n.d.

Sources: CDC, National Center for Health Statistics, *National Health and Nutrition Examination Survey: Health, United States* (2002), http://www.cdc.gov/nchs/products/pubs/pubd/hestats/obese/obse99.htm; Flegal et al., *JAMA* 288 (2002): 1723–27; NIH, National Heart, Lung, and Blood Institute, *Clinical Guidelines on the Identification, Evaluation and Treatment of Overweight and Obesity in Adults* (1998), http://hp2010.nhlbihin.net/oei_ss/download/pdf/CORESET1.pdf.

Olshansky and colleagues proposed that the obesity epidemic may even threaten the nearly 170-year-long trend of increasing life expectancy.[25] According to Kenneth Thorpe, obesity-related illnesses also accounted for 27 percent of the inflation-adjusted increase in the cost of health care from 1987 to 2002 and may outstrip smoking as the most costly behavioral health risk.[26]

A recent University of Pennsylvania study suggested that older baby boomers have lower self-reported health status than a previous generation reported twelve years earlier, for reasons that appear at least circumstantially to be related to obesity. For example, 22 percent of "early" boomer men and 33 percent of "early" boomer women reported difficulty getting out of a chair, nearly double the percentages of the same age cohort sampled twelve years earlier.

Recently, however, analysis of data on mortality trends among Americans of various weights have cast doubt on the seemingly overpowering evidence of the effect of obesity on mortality risk.[27] Analysis by Katherine Flegal for the Centers for Disease Control undercut earlier estimates of 300,000 deaths per year from obesity, which were derived from 1970 health data, by suggesting that recent advances, particularly in cardiac care, may have markedly reduced health risks for obese people. Flegal also found those who are merely overweight, who outnumber the obese, may live longer than those of normal or slightly below-normal weight.[28]

It is difficult to reconcile the easy correlation between obesity and, particularly, cardiac risk with the remarkably durable and apparently accelerating downtrend in death rates from heart disease shown in figure 4.1. Management of the more proximate risk factors of heart disease (namely, high LDL cholesterol and hypertension) may enable larger numbers of obese people to survive some of the more lethal correlates of obesity, though at a significant cost in prescription medication.

Olshanky's research also found that the greatest mortality risk from obesity falls on the young and middle aged. This result was confirmed by a more recent Rand Corporation study, which reported that those obese individuals who survive to Medicare age live about as long as their nonobese peers, although with 34 percent higher lifetime medical costs.[29]

So catastropharian accountants will have to subtract the Social Security and Medicare revenues that younger obese persons who do not live long enough to collect from those obesity-related expenses and "return" the funds to the federal treasury. Although obesity will challenge the quality of life for many baby boomers, its long-term economic impact is still unclear. It is also not clear that the prevalence of obesity among Americans cannot be slowed or reversed by changing social values, public health awareness, and improved health benefit design that encourages exercise and weight loss. Trend is not necessarily destiny.

Alzheimer's Disease: A More Serious Threat

A more serious cause for concern may be the potential impact of Alzheimer's disease. The death of Ronald Reagan in 2004 from complications of Alzheimer's disease raised the profile of this dreadful illness, which afflicts many millions of older Americans. Some 47 percent of those over age 85 have symptoms of this chronic degenerative disease of the nervous system.[30] Currently, the only way to diagnose this condition definitively is at autopsy.

Alzheimer's disease destroys a person's memory, personality, and capacity for self-management. The disease is progressive and incurable. By the time it has run its course, the person must be either in-stitutionalized or under twenty-four-hour caregiver supervision in the home. Present medications for the disease slow its progression only modestly. The potential of Alzheimer's disease to incapacitate a large number of baby boomers is very real. According to the Alzheimer's Association, the prevalence of Alzheimer's disease among the nation's older citizens is increasing: an estimated 4.5 million Americans currently have Alzheimer's disease. The number of Americans with Alzheimer's disease has more than doubled since 1980 and will continue to grow: by 2050 the number of individuals with Alzheimer's disease could range from 11.3 million to 16 million.[31] This number would actually be increased by medical successes against other diseases, such as heart disease, cancer, and stroke, because they enable individuals to survive long enough to develop Alzheimer's.

Finding a cure for Alzheimer's disease, or a method of replacing damaged nervous system tissues, is a particularly strategic scientific goal, given its disproportionate potential for improving the health status of older Americans. As with another degenerative nervous system illness, Parkinson's disease, scientific progress in understanding Alzheimer's disease has been painfully slow. With the benefit of hindsight, for baby boomers, the "Decade of the Brain," a disappointing federal brain research initiative launched by the National Institutes of Health in 1990, should have been the 1980s.

Some recent research, however, has suggested that the widespread phenomenon of short-term memory loss may be attributable not to Alzheimer's disease but to the cumulative effect of silent "ministrokes" and vascular system failures that limit blood supply to brain tissues.[32] By destroying brain tissues, these barely detectable ministrokes impair the ability of the brain to consolidate and retrieve memories.

The fact that some memory loss associated with aging may have vascular, rather than nervous system, origins provides some hope that improved management of the risks for vascular disease, particularly controlling high blood pressure and cholesterol levels, will have as a collateral benefit the improvement of cognitive functioning of older people. A possible unforeseen by-product of the steady increase in the use of statin drugs and efforts by people to reduce cholesterol intake in their diets may be reductions in damaging vascular events in the brain, thus preserving memory capacity. The scientific evidence of any effect from statin use in prevention of Alzheimer's disease is equivocal.[33]

Alzheimer's disease is a crushing burden on the families of persons with the disease today. From a societal standpoint, the risks from Alzheimer's disease and other degenerative diseases of the nervous and musculoskeletal system ramp up aggressively in the decade of 2030 and after, when the first baby boomers reach their 80s. No scientific advance would have a more positive effect on the ultimate health prospects of the baby boom than finding a cure for this dread disease.

The Most Serious Health Risks for Baby Boomers Are Twenty Years Away

The prospects for healthy aging will materially improve the outlook for the baby boom generation. However, these improvements and the benefits to individuals and society will not happen by themselves. Without active efforts by policy makers, employers, the medical care system, and boomers themselves, the full economic and human potential of improved health in aging will not be realized. To achieve them, we must shed the idea that isolation, dependency, and rapid declines in cognitive and physical capacity, among older Americans are somehow biologically inevitable. They are not.

If we could articulate a single health policy objective for older Americans, it would be to do everything possible to extend their functional life-span. No one has articulated the steps needed to achieve this better than Rowe and Kahn in *Successful Aging*. Manton's positive trend seems likely to continue, reinforced by the emerging clinical tool set and the opportunities embodied in life-style, diet, and other changes people can make themselves to improve health. Improving health among older people, as well as the behavioral potential for significant further improvements, not only will facilitate a more active and productive later life course for baby boomers but also will alleviate the near-term health care cost and dependency burden on baby boomers' families.

The recent studies suggesting that early baby boomers might have, on average, somewhat lower health status than their age peers twelve years earlier should concern us. The University of Pennsylvania's researchers found that "a large group of the respondents aged 51–56 reports few chronic conditions, little pain, no restrictions in activity or cognitive problems. But a small fraction is in very poor health, with multiple chronic conditions, regular and severe pain, or moderate cognitive impairment."[34] The health problems of this small fraction are significant enough to affect the group's averages. This finding supports the baby boomer segmentation scheme proposed in the preceding chapter and validates the policy goal of focusing earlier and more aggressively on the health problems of the so-called Struggling and Anxious baby boomers.

No matter how much scientific progress we make between now and then, the period from 2030 to 2050 is likely to be expensive for American society. Many of the measures I discuss in subsequent chapters will be needed to avoid significant fiscal dislocation in those two decades. Making the most of the next twenty-plus years—in reforming health care payment, encouraging healthier aging, making meaningful scientific progress in understanding and controlling chronic disease, and continuing to grow the U.S. economy—will be essential for creating the fiscal and social capacity to absorb the ultimate health care costs of the baby boomers.

Changing health insurance, employment policy, tax policy, and legal protections for older workers holds the potential for averting the catastropharian scenario and creating assets on the social balance sheet to counterbalance the inevitable rising liabilities of an older population. The rest of this book explores the options to leverage the positive trends in a longer productive work life and healthier aging for baby boomers through a pro-work, health-sustaining social policy.

five

Encouraging Work in Later Life

What Can Be Done?

The U.S. economy generates more than 30 percent of the world's wealth. But is it possible for even a wealthy society to finance an entitlement to a work-free twenty-plus-year period at the end of a twenty-first-century worker's life? Given the advances in life expectancy and functional life-spans that have taken place during the past eighty years, it is difficult to defend the idea that age 65 should continue to be the pivot point for public policy toward older Americans.

It appears that baby boomers expect to continue working longer and in far larger numbers than their parents' or grandparents' generations. Further, many more of them will be healthy enough to sustain longer work careers. Finally, there is clear evidence of a looming shortage, particularly, of skilled workers, in coming decades. These facts beg an important question: what can we do to enable or actively encourage longer work careers? We must not only consider some creative solutions to the problem but also deal with some of the constraints that prevent modernizing our work force policies to take these new realities into account.

Today, the public cost of removing workers from the labor market at or before age 65 is being financed by deficit spending, which is financed by selling U.S. Treasury securities in large part to non-Americans. Many of the largest purchasers, notably China and Japan, will have far larger problems supporting their aging populations than we will and are unlikely sources of future largess. Corporations finance retirement costs by invading current cash flow, displacing investment in new technology and creation of new jobs, and, if they fail, shifting those costs onto the government.

The popular press is replete with stories of the thinning of the retirement safety net for Americans. Employers are struggling under the burden of retiree health and pension costs and have been shedding these responsibilities. Confrontations have multiplied in the past decade within troubled mature industries such as the legacy airlines, steel, and domestic auto makers over the cost of retirement promises made during the boom years of the 1950s and 1960s. Present fiscal and corporate retirement policies are clearly not sustainable.

The real question is *how* to change them. Instead of tilting older workers toward an early and heavily subsidized exit from labor markets, and penalizing those who continue working, as present Social Security and tax policies do, can we find mechanisms to actively encourage longer, and/or multiple, work careers for older workers and a more seamless relationship among compensation, savings, and retirement benefits?

The Increasingly Virtual Workplace

A sensible employment policy should recognize that today's work force is engaged in fundamentally different work from that of the boomers' parents and grandparents. There is still backbreaking and dangerous manual labor in our economy. People still harvest timber from mountainsides and pull fish from the Gulf of Alaska. They still make steel and restring high-tension wires 100 feet above the ground. They still work on automobile assembly lines and connect the steel beams on skyscrapers. But these workers are increasingly rare. Less than 8 percent of the contemporary U.S. work force engages in physically strenuous work, compared to 20 percent in 1950 (figure 5.1).

Not that we produce less food or manufactured goods than sixty years ago. On the contrary, extraordinary advances in productivity

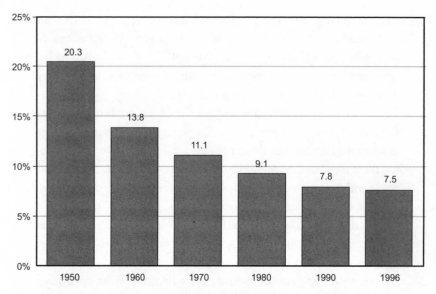

Figure 5.1. U.S. workers in physically demanding jobs, 1950–1996
Source: Urban Institute, Washington, D.C., 1999.

and a global economy have dramatically reduced the number of people required to create these goods for us and have lowered the cost in real dollars (as well as the amount of energy required) to create the material foundation of modern life.

The modern economy is, as Peter Drucker first observed, a knowledge economy whose core products are not physical goods but intellectual property. Today's workers are increasingly knowledge workers, who work at desks and computer terminals both to create new knowledge and to employ that knowledge to create value, or service workers, who create value by interacting with us.

The leading edge of this new economy is the knowledge worker. Knowledge workers write software, novels, and screenplays. They teach kindergartners and graduate students. They write laws and legal briefs. They develop new medicines and technology for diagnosing illness. They write product specifications and technical manuals. They design homes, factories, office complexes, and public infrastructure. They create new computer chips and the software and information architectures that animate them. In short, they create new intellectual property.

Robert Reich, in *Work of Nations,* called these knowledge workers "symbolic analysts."[1] Richard Florida termed them "the creative class."[2] Florida estimates that this group accounts for 30 percent of the employment in the U.S. economy and 47 percent of all salary and wages paid. Although we no longer manufacture much of what we consume, the United States dominates the rest of the world in the creation of new intellectual property.[3]

The new scientific and technical knowledge that forms the foundation of modern manufacturing is made in the United States. Though other countries are catching up, the United States leads the world in new patents filed and new software code written.[4] On a nation-by-nation basis, the long-standing U.S. scientific dominance continues, though other areas of the world are rapidly closing the gap.[5]

The modern U.S. economy is not only a knowledge economy but also a service economy. Service workers help us rehabilitate ourselves from strokes or sports injuries. They help us plan for and invest our wealth. They massage our bodies and style our hair. They prepare and serve us food and help us carry it to our waiting minivans. They repair damaged heart valves and replace worn-out joints. They sell us clothing and life insurance policies. They help us manage our money and help corporations decide where to put their capital. The most dynamic sector of the U.S. economy, the health care system, combines knowledge and service workers in its 16-million-person work force.[6]

The Emergence of the Free Agent

The rise of the "creative class" has coincided with the emergence of a flexible free-agent work force, in which talent migrates from larger firms to boutique-type firms or self-employment. Talent and relationships inhere not in corporations but in individuals, in what they know and whom they connect to. Nearly all the job growth in the economy in the past twenty years has been from small firms and sole proprietorships. In 2000–2001, a period of mild recession, small businesses created all of the net new jobs in the United States. Firms with fewer than 500 employees saw a net increase in employment of 1,150,875; at the same time, large-business employment decreased by 150,905.[7] The small-business share varies from year to year and reflects economic trends. Over the decade of the 1990s, small-business net job creation fluctuated between 60 and 80 percent of total new jobs.[8] Having small businesses account for all of the net new jobs is not unique to 2000–2001; during an economic downturn in the early 1990s, a similar result occurred.[9]

Knowledge workers increasingly work for themselves. More than 16 million Americans are self-employed, a growth rate of 5.7 percent from 2002 to 2003.[10] Almost 25 percent of those workers over age 50 are self-employed. According to WorldatWork, 20 percent of the U.S. work force engages in telework. Broadband use has dramatically expanded this practice, with the number of broadband-enabled teleworkers rising to 19.1 million in 2006.[11]

This number seems poised to double in the next ten years, as more businesses take advantage of broadband connectivity and new business tools to connect workers to customers and colleagues from home. According to a survey by Booz Allen Hamilton, not only is home sourcing cheaper than traditional outsourcing, but home agents are also 25 percent more productive than employees who manage calls in-house.[12] About 20 percent of all customer service call-center agents in the United States now take calls from their homes. Office Depot closed ten of its twelve call centers this year, replacing nearly 1,000 full-time agents with home-based ones.[13] According to a recent study done for the Consumer Electronics Association, telecommuting also saved 840 million gallons of gas a year, reducing greenhouse gas emissions by nearly 14 million metric tons.[14]

Thanks to the Internet, knowledge creation can take place anywhere the knowledge worker is and anywhere he or she can gain access to databases and the opinions and input of others. Working from home has been a particularly salient trend in large metropolitan areas such as Los Angeles, Washington, D.C., Seattle, and Boston, where surface transportation networks may be in gridlock twelve or more hours a day. In southern California, nearly 23 percent of telecommuters are in their 50s, compared with only 16.7 percent overall and less than 16 percent of nonteleworkers.[15]

The ability of knowledge workers to share work projects from different locations has been made possible by the development of "groupware." Lotus Notes was an early example. Groove Network's products are a more recent, broadband-enabled example. Groove, which was recently acquired by Microsoft, is a peer-to-peer networking tool set. Groove Workspaces serve as virtual offices, in which geographically dispersed co-workers can store files and folders, save threaded discussions, share calendars, track project information and timelines, meet online, share a whiteboard, and communicate through chat and instant messaging. Google has developed a similar set of groupware applications.

The growth and increasing integration of conferencing software into the computer desktop has enabled video teleconferencing to be launched off a button on the Web browser, as in Microsoft's Live-Meeting and Apple's iChat. With colleagues working in different time zones, it is becoming more difficult for co-workers to meet face to face, making the use of such conferencing software much more common. Groupware and affordable videoconferencing enabled by broadband Internet connection has enabled asynchronous, multisite teams to assemble around particular tasks, disband, and reform around new tasks.

As broadband has become ubiquitous, knowledge work is rapidly becoming a truly global activity. "Nighthawk" radiologists can read magnetic resonance imaging (MRI) scans a half a world away, while those who captured the images are sleeping, and can communicate their interpretations to the physicians who ordered the test asynchronously. Intensive-care physicians can monitor gravely ill patients in as many as five distinct locations from a console that provides video feeds, live audio links to the on-site care team, and a dashboard of real-time clinical indicators, care pathways, alerts, and predictive tools for each patient.[16]

Software engineers and coders can produce software literally twenty-four hours a day in teams separated geographically by 10,000 miles but working from common architectures and an integrated work plan. Global information networks can speed the fulfillment of orders and the processing of claims and bills. Scientific teams can write and edit papers around the clock, with data, exhibits, and comments flowing continuously from author to author.

Technological advances have created opportunities for workers to operate from anywhere and to craft work schedules to fit around family obligations and recreational interests. They will also accelerate the already robust trend toward free agency and self-employment among workers. Though associated with younger workers, these trends will transform the work careers and lives of older workers and facilitate a sharp increase in older workers' labor force participation in coming years. Airline reservationists working in bunny slippers in their living rooms can book our reservations, as JetBlue's reservationists do. Many of JetBlue's living room reservation cadres are "retirees" from other industries or government.

This progress has come at a steep price: the abolition of the bright line between work and leisure. The "office" is already less and less a place that we visit and increasingly something we carry in our pocket. Work has become a state of being that begins when we switch on a wireless device. Whether it is on ski lifts, on beaches, and even on horseback or bicycles (!), ubiquitous access to communications networks (through Blackberries or multifunction cell phones) has virtually obliterated the notion of pure leisure. Most boomers will have worked with and learned how to use these tools long before they reach conventional retirement age. Younger knowledge workers will never know that there used to be hard physical boundaries between work and leisure.

Implications for the Older Worker

The emergence of a real-time, networked, knowledge-based economy has important implications for older workers. As workers age, their store of knowledge and the breadth of their personal networks both grow and become more valuable. Many older workers in law, medicine, engineering, sales and marketing, management consulting, and other fields may well be worth more than their less-experienced younger colleagues, even if productivity and intellectual flexibility may tail off toward the end of the work career.

As knowledge work has replaced back-breaking physical labor and mind-numbing factory assembly-line work, the capacity of workers to have longer careers has increased apace. Combine this with the increasing comfort workers have in mobility among firms and even among careers, and we have not only the recipe for a more flexible and adaptable labor market but also the potential for fulfilling, serial careers. As Dychtwald and others have long predicted, this pattern will define career paths for many baby boomers over the next twenty-plus years.

These changes reinforce the pattern of increased worker independence and labor mobility seen among baby boom workers. Boomers pioneered the institution of free agency—in sports and in business. Free agency fit the high autonomy needs and antibureaucratic values of boomers, and it also met the economy's need for a more flexible and deployable work force. Employers of knowledge workers turned to contracting and outsourcing for more of their work products not only for relief from long-term benefits commitments but also, and perhaps more so, for the ability to staff projects, start up new ventures, and organize around product launches more quickly, more efficiently, and flexibly.

Encouraging Longer Work Careers

The appropriate response to tightening skilled labor markets and the soaring cost of retiree benefits is to make fewer retirees or to create them at a far slower pace. So the urgent question for employers is how to switch gears and both retain and cultivate their older workers.

The concept of retirement as a sharply demarcated transition from full-time work to full-time leisure will be replaced by a more gradual, flexible, and thoughtfully supported transition from full-time work. Some baby boomers may indeed elect the abrupt cessation of work characterized by earlier retirement models, but many more will opt for phased retirement, while others will sustain the

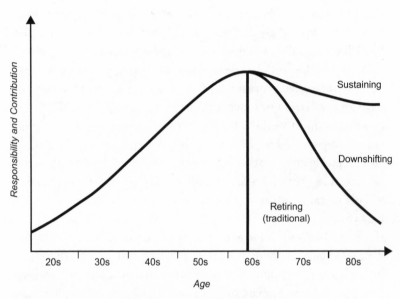

Figure 5.2. Three career trajectories
Source: Ken Dychtwald, *Workforce Crisis* (Boston: Harvard Business School Press, 2006).

pace of work with only a modest diminution of effort until the end of their lives (figure 5.2).

Lots of things can be done to encourage longer and more diverse career paths. They include ending mandatory retirement policies, improving worker performance evaluation and compensation schemes, creating new and more flexible work roles, reducing the economic burdens associated with self-employment, revising pension and health benefits policies to support those new work roles, and helping encourage the formation of retirement capital to support both future incomes and health benefits.

To support new career trajectories for older workers will require not only creativity on the part of employers but also changes in the Internal Revenue Code and the Employee Retirement Income Security Act (ERISA), as well as in the Age Discrimination in Employment Act (ADEA), enacted in 1967 to protect older workers from job discrimination. These legal provisions form a dense web of restrictions on employer conduct that date from the end of the industrial era and that fundamentally constrain those who wish to retain or repurpose their older workers.[17]

Mandatory retirement policies were used for decades as a way of assuring the renewal of the work force and creating employment opportunities inside firms for younger workers. These are not inherently unworthy objectives. However, they also served corporate interests, because they enabled firms to replace workers who had high salaries and benefits costs with younger, healthier, lower-wage workers.

Mandatory retirement programs served as a nonjudgmental device for separating less-effective older workers from their jobs. Instead of risking lawsuits by directly challenging or terminating ineffective or unproductive workers, employers could simply let nature do the dirty work for them. Most mandatory retirement policies were prohibited in 1978 by the Age Discrimination in Employment Act, with phased elimination of mandatory retirement for tenured workers, such as college professors, by 1993.[18] However, less-formal methods than mandatory retirement still push older workers from the workplace by diminishing their pension benefits or restricting their mobility through up-or-out promotion policy.

Despite these legal protections embodied in ADEA, many corporate human resource managers continue to view the older worker as a cost burden. In many cases, this is simply a function of shoddy cost analysis. While it is simple to quantify the higher salary and benefits expenses of older workers, it is easy to underestimate the cost of training replacements and the lower productivity of younger workers.

For example, the hypothetical salary of a medical or surgical nurse may be $46,832, but the cost of replacing that nurse with an inexperienced younger worker is estimated at between $92,442 and $145,000. These costs include advertising and interviewing, overtime, temporary replacement costs, and lost productivity.[19] If a hospital with 100 nurses experienced turnover at the national average rate of 21.3 percent, these expenditures could amount to almost $2 million yearly.[20] A recent study by Towers Perrin, a corporate benefits consultant, estimated that the total cost of doubling the number of new nursing hires over age 55 (from 20% to 40% of new hires) would be 1 percent per employee.[21]

Replacement costs for skilled workers are mounting rapidly, as extraordinary recruitment expenses, including generous relocation allowances, signing bonuses, sharply higher base wages, and other inducements have dramatically increased the expense of replacing older workers. As labor markets tighten, employers will discover that the competition for younger workers will raise their wage and salary expenses and require more generous health insurance coverage than when they had long lines of younger baby boomers waiting for work.

In the absence of mandatory retirement, employers will have to create performance-evaluation tools and systems to more rigorously evaluate the productivity of its entire work force. Rather than allowing retirement policies to sweep all workers out of their firms at an arbitrary age, employers will have to deal honestly with the large variation in worker productivity and quality and to create defensible mechanisms for separating the less-effective older workers from employment, while retaining and investing in the more-productive ones.

More rigorous evaluation of older workers and firing or retraining unproductive workers for cause may create legal liability for employers under ADEA. This statute also constrains employers who wish to offer older workers health insurance options different from those for younger workers. The legal issues here are complex and beyond the scope of this book. Finding the appropriate balance between protecting older workers from age discrimination and permitting firms to selectively extend the work careers of their best older workers is going to challenge both the corporate human resources community and lawmakers.

Flexible Careers, Flexible Retirement

The major challenge in retaining older workers is in reshaping work roles to accommodate the reality that they may wish a different blending of work and leisure from that offered to younger workers. Many organizations that struggled with worker shortages during the late 1980s and early 1990s experimented with flexible work schedules to attract or retain younger employees. Hospitals were forced to create more flexible work assignments to minimize their contracting out for nurses and bring their salary expenses back under control. Hospitals that used temporary staffing agencies paid as much as double the conventional salaries of employed nurses and technicians.[22]

These flexible work arrangements that include variable-day and variable-week schedules that usually require a specified number of hours per pay period are frequently grouped under the umbrella term *flextime*.[23] The most popular flexible work schedules included three twelve-hour shifts followed by four days off; rotation among day, swing, and evening shifts in four-month intervals; two weeks on and two weeks off; and four ten-hour days, with one day off a week. Shared employment, or "job sharing," is also an enticing form of flexible scheduling for career-oriented nurses. This arrangement is especially attractive to those who wish to remain in the work force but need to work part time temporarily to attend to family responsibilities.[24]

For older workers, different types of flexibility may be needed, including task- or project-oriented work (as is typical in consulting, software development, or entertainment industries such as motion pictures or recording); six months on and six months off (for workers with vacation homes in sunny or snowy climates); asynchronous work scheduling, in which tasks accumulate in the computer inbox to be completed as time becomes available; or simply traditional part-time work roles requiring commitments of two or three days a week. Home Depot offers its older workers an innovative "snowbird special," in which they can work winters in Florida and summers in stores in Maine or elsewhere in the northeast.[25]

New work roles are also emerging for older workers, patterned on the professor emeritus designation in college and university faculties. These roles permit part-time employment with continued full-time benefits, in which the older worker mentors or trains younger associates, participates in governance activities, or performs community trusteeship or volunteer work on behalf of the employer. The person can also function as an internal trustee or keeper of corporate lore and traditions as a senior member of project teams or divisions, who can edit and evaluate work products produced by those teams.

Deloitte Consulting created a senior leaders program to retain experienced consulting partners, who were encouraged to design second careers with the firm with flexible hours in new locations.[26]

Bon Secours Health System, in Richmond, Virginia, a Catholic multihospital system, has made reshaping the work roles of its older workers a major priority and has been rewarded by a high listing among AARP's 50 Best Employers for Workers over 50. More than 30 percent of Bon Secours's largely female work force is over age 50. The hospital system offered older workers full benefits for fifteen or more hours a week, or an opt-out for higher wages for those on Medicare or with a spouse's health coverage. It enabled older workers to switch freely from full-time to part-time to on-call status according to their own needs and schedules without interrupting benefits. It also provided senior-oriented wellness services and both child and older adult day care.[27]

A major issue for many older workers who desire a flexible retirement is using their pension assets to smooth over cash needs during the periods they do not work. Those older workers who wish to accept a work schedule of six months on and six months off or part-time employment were, until recently, forbidden from accessing their pension balances to support them during "off" periods, because they could not collect their pensions until after they completely ceased working. Some firms attempted to work around these restrictions by permitting workers to retire and then rehiring them part time after a waiting period.

IRS rule changes in 2004 enabled people to access their pensions without penalty if they reduce their work schedules 20 percent below full-time levels, while continuing to accrue pension benefits for the hours they do work.[28] Workers must be at least age $59\frac{1}{2}$ to be eligible. Older workers for whom continued corporate health benefits are as important as or more important than salary find their benefits threatened if they reduce their work schedules below a certain number of hours. Employers who wish to offer older workers a different health benefits package from younger workers find themselves constrained by ADEA.

Many firms have begun this process of culture change, but the process needs to be accelerated. As late as 2001, only about one-fifth of the nation's employers offered a phased retirement option to their older workers.[29] Older organizations are the first to feel the impact of this knowledge loss, as they lose experienced employees, which is one reason why public universities were quick to embrace this trend. In 1998 the University of North Carolina began a pilot phased retirement program allowing faculty members over the age of 50 to work half time at half salary for up to three years while collecting partial pension benefits. Today, almost one-third of retiring faculty members at the sixteen UNC campuses take advantage of phased retirement, and the concept is slowly spreading to many other public and private organizations.[30]

One of the most important constraints on the adoption of more flexible work arrangements is defined-benefit pension plans. Older workers who accept lower salaries in exchange for a flexible work schedule may find their pension benefits reduced if they were based on their final-year salary. A typical plan may set the normal retirement age at 65, but a worker who started at age 25 is likely to find that the expected value of the pension accrues most rapidly between ages 51 and 55 under reasonable economic assumptions. Soon after 55, the accrual might turn negative, reducing the ultimate payout for each additional year worked. That is to say, the increased pension earned by working an extra year does not compensate for the fact that the person will receive one less year of benefits.[31]

To address this problem, firms have switched from defined contribution pensions to defined benefit or cash balance plans that calculate retirement plan contributions in a fixed percentage of salary regardless of age.[32] The ability to make these changes is constrained for many older firms and public-sector employers by union collective bargaining agreements.

Health Insurance: The Largest Barrier

Health care costs create a daunting barrier to hiring or retaining older workers. The premium for a standard health insurance policy for 55- to 59-year-olds can be more than double that for 20- to 44-year-olds. Phased retirees may end up not receiving health insurance coverage or being asked to pay higher employee co-insurance, as well as sacrificing life or disability insurance coverage, or accepting less paid vacation time.[33]

In the not-too-distant future, older workers who are self-employed, independent contractors, or consultants may outnumber older workers in salaried employment. Daunting challenges await those whose career paths take them into self-employment or the creation of new enterprises later in life. By far the most significant challenge for those who become self-employed before reaching the age of eligibility for Medicare is finding affordable health insurance coverage. Health coverage for workers who are 50-plus is not optional; given the health risks of later middle age, it is vital.

Until they reach the age of eligibility for Medicare, older workers may discover that individual health insurance coverage is prohibitively expensive or simply not available from any carrier. Competition among health insurance providers in the individual market is typically far thinner than for small or medium-sized firms. Health insurers are reluctant to cover older workers as individuals; a 60-year-old worker can reliably be expected to generate fully triple the annual health expense of a 40-year-old worker![34]

The expected revolution in access to affordable health insurance through Internet purchasing pools has yet to materialize, despite the fact that other industries, such as travel, auto insurance, and personal computing, have been able to use Internet utilities and call centers to enable sophisticated customization of purchases by individuals and companies. These innovations have brought corporate purchasing clout to individuals through competitive Web sites such as Expedia, Travelocity, and Hotels.com.

Congress has struggled for nearly a decade without success to solve this problem by encouraging multiple-employer pooled purchasing of health insurance. Some organizations, such as professional associations, have successfully enabled their free-agent members to purchase health insurance coverage at levels approximating group rates. However, more comprehensive legislative reforms enabling larger numbers of "free agents" to pool their health insurance purchasing power have been blocked by the politically powerful independent insurance brokers, who control access to individual and small group insurance markets. Recent congressional experiments with "multiple employer welfare arrangements," or MEWAs, ended in a rash of bankrupt health insurance trusts and fraud investigations.

One possible solution, which a group of the human resource directors of large corporations are exploring, is using their corporations' purchasing leverage to offer grouplike health insurance rates to their independent contractors, to be purchased with their own resources. National Health Access, consisting of a large group of employers and three major health insurers, has launched a program that enables part-time workers as well as independent contractors to receive access to new health coverage options. Participating companies are using their purchasing power to obtain insurance rates and terms that are more favorable than what workers would obtain individually.[35]

Another innovative approach to covering free agents is the New York–based "freelancers union" for self-employed workers called Working Today.[36] Working Today, which had 56,000 members as of the fall of 2007, enables freelance workers to obtain affordable health insurance, disability insurance, and other benefits at group rates. The group also facilitates online linkages to exchange work opportunities and face-to-face networking among its members through Meetup. The group's logo, appropriately enough, is bees buzzing around a hive.

Earlier Access to Medicare?

Medicare was originally created to solve a problem of access to health insurance by older Americans. Several possible Medicare policy changes, which are discussed at greater length in chapter 6, might markedly improve access to health insurance for older workers, enabling longer work careers.

One possibility, advocated by Rudolph Penner and colleagues at the Urban Institute, is to eliminate the requirement, enacted in 1982, that Medicare be a secondary payer for employees over age 65 who are also covered by a private health plan. This would also address the

inequity that employed people over age 65 are denied access to benefits they have been paying for all their working lives *because they are*
working. This policy change would alleviate an economic burden on
employers and create an incentive to keep people working after age
65, though at some cost to the federal budget.[37]

Another possible solution, which surfaced during the 2004 presidential campaign, is permitting older workers who have trouble obtaining affordable health insurance coverage to buy into Medicare
after age 55, paying the premiums out of pocket as individuals, or receiving them as a benefit from their employer. Medicare premiums
would be adjusted to reflect the lower age and severity of illness of the
younger, still-working population. Self-employed individuals would
benefit by having access to a federal health program with low administrative expenses and broad provider networks and cost controls.

This idea would leverage existing payment arrangements between
the Medicare program and virtually all of the hospitals and physicians that Medicare reaches. It would add younger workers and a
flow of voluntary contributions to the Medicare program. A broader
enrollment base might deter some health care providers, particularly
specialty physicians, from closing their practices to Medicare beneficiaries.

A more private-sector-oriented approach would be to permit self-
employed people to buy into the Federal Employees Health Benefits
Program (FEHBP), which relies on private health plans to cover federal workers. FEHBP has significant influence with private health
plans, particularly in areas with large numbers of federal workers,
and it provides a modern, multiple-choice health benefits alternative
that leverages the influence of the private health plan market on
providers.

Ending Employer-Based Health Insurance?

These approaches beg a larger question, however. How sensible is
it to continue using an employer-based health benefits model to provide health coverage? Employer-based insurance emerged during
World War II from the single-firm, one-career manufacturing econ-

omy. It has served as a powerful device for reducing worker mobility. Maximizing worker mobility will help keep knowledge workers in the work force longer and reduce burnout, poor morale, and other symptoms of a trapped work force. Employer-based insurance may be an idea whose time is passing.

Disconnecting the health benefit from employment is probably the best long-term approach for an emerging knowledge economy. Finding a tax-based method of offering health insurance vouchers directly to individuals would be a better way to achieve change in work roles than continuing the present tax code's rich subsidies to employer-based insurance, whose present costs are estimated at $140 billion a year.[38] Senator Ron Wyden recently introduced a proposal for national health insurance based on this idea.[39]

In a tax-based approach, working people would be required to purchase health insurance for themselves, and those with incomes below a certain threshold would receive subsidies in the form of refundable tax credits to enable that purchase. Employers would be required to pass the money they formerly spent on worker health benefits through to workers' paychecks. It is worth noting that the cost of subsidizing older persons' purchase of individual health insurance would be prohibitive unless some way could be found to pool their purchasing power and to protect them from underwriting based on preexisting conditions.

Such an approach to universal health insurance was offered fifteen years ago by the libertarian Heritage Foundation during the debate over the ill-fated Clinton health reforms. Economist Victor Fuchs recently offered such an idea as a model for universal health insurance, with the vouchers funded by a national value-added tax.[40] The state of Massachusetts recently enacted a mixed model, which preserved employer-based insurance, combining an employer mandate to purchase insurance for workers for all firms of more than fifty employees with an individual mandate that individuals purchase health insurance or face higher state income taxes.[41] Massachusetts also created a health care purchasing intermediary to obtain affordable coverage for individuals. The effectiveness of these reforms remains to be evaluated.

The daunting hurdle facing those who want to replace employer-based insurance with individual-based insurance is the fact that employers are currently voluntarily paying some $700 billion in private insurance premiums (supported by the aforementioned $140 billion in tax exemptions). To replace these premium flows with federal revenues would require finding new tax dollars in a political climate both lacking in trust and fiercely hostile to new tax levies for any purpose. Whether employers favor surrendering control over the health benefit and supporting a new tax to alleviate their health benefits costs will probably be determined by the intensity of the next surge in health insurance costs.

Employer Help in Rewiring

Another important way in which employers can help retain older workers is assisting them in retraining and developing skills that permit them to move laterally in the organization, or helping them move into administrative roles that leverage their knowledge of the organization's history and values. Typically, employers reserve their training budget for younger workers. However, restricting training and work force development programs to younger workers has hampered employers' ability to increase the flexibility with which it can deploy older workers. Human resource managers should assume that a subset of their workers could remain employed into their 70s, and they should approach the training and development of 50- and 60-year-old workers on that basis. Managers should be provided with special training to handle age extremes, when peers or subordinates are much older or younger.[42] Workers of all ages should be supported with technology, in addition to face-to-face time.[43]

Achenbaum suggested an innovative idea for funding the retraining of older workers: permitting them to borrow against their accumulated equity in Social Security funds "to pay for training that will enhance their worth and longevity in the labor force."[44] This idea would disconnect access to late-career training and development from the employer, as well as provide the self-employed in lower-income bands access to funding that enabled them to move laterally in the economy.

More-Accessible Information Technology

One area of particular importance in the training and development of older workers is assuring that many of these workers, who spent the majority of their work career in the predigital age, have the computer skills needed to take advantage of the networked, real-time workplace. Younger workers, whose computer skills came to them in childhood, take to new computing applications, manipulation of databases, multilateral and continuous messaging, and complex searches as naturally as breathing. They learned to use computers, literally, by playing with them. Older workers, many of whom have lost their playfulness, continue to struggle with learning and applying computer applications to their work.

Employers can fill a critical gap by creating computer-skills-enhancement programs for their older workers. Many older workers are reluctant to admit they need the help, but employers should make them available nonetheless. Improving older workers' computer skills will pay off many times over in improved productivity and increased capacity to work in decentralized, asynchronous team settings. Teaching older workers search skills and enabling them to network with colleagues in other firms in parallel functional disciplines will also enhance their value as employees or later as contractors or consultants.

Software vendors can make a measurable contribution by investing in improving usability. Part of what held down the adoption of computer skills by people older than 40 was the need to learn a private language of commands and utilities to perform vital computing functions. The weedlike proliferation of features and functions in business software has been a daunting barrier to adoption for older workers.

More-intuitive and better-designed user interfaces will help. Business and personal software will come to market in the next few years with the ability to customize what is presented to the user based on his or her work style, work flows, and past knowledge-seeking behavior.[45] Computer systems will dramatically increase their "intelligence" in years ahead, and much of the advance will enable customization of functions to the individual needs and styles of specific users, young or old.

Eventually software will play a key role in teaching workers of all ages more about their businesses, by seeking out and archiving knowledge the worker may not even know existed and by sensing the need for specific knowledge in normal workflow. This is likely to be especially important in knowledge-intensive fields such as law, medicine, and engineering, in which knowledge-management practices have often not kept pace with the flood of new knowledge.

Personal Plans, Social Benefits

It is difficult to overstate how much of a difference encouraging older workers to continue to work will have in averting the catastropharian scenario. *Business Week* recently estimated that increased productivity of older workers, when combined with higher labor force participation rates of baby boomers, could add 9 percent to U.S. GDP by 2045—in today's dollars, an additional $3 trillion.[46]

Facilitating longer work careers by baby boomers will not only create wealth but also make it possible for many boomers to defer receiving public benefits until they decide to stop working. The fiscal consequences are not inconsiderable. When a $50,000-a-year worker retires, not only does national income decline by $50,000, but also the retired worker's costs shift onto the rest of society in the form of $23,500 in Social Security and Medicare benefits. Governments also lose $18,300 in taxes because there are no longer wages and salary to tax, for a net shift to society of $41,800 for each year.[47]

These estimates do not take into account the effect on the society's health care costs of postponing increased morbidity associated with retirement, which was discussed earlier. Working longer will pay huge dividends not only for boomers but for the nation's struggling Social Security system. A recent Urban Institute study found that working five more years could not only increase workers' lifetime income after age fifty by 56% but generate enough additional tax revenues (Social Security and federal income tax) to close the Social Security funding deficit, discussed in Chapter 7.[48] Postponing retirement creates tremendous fiscal leverage by creating income in place of societal outlays. In intergenerational accounting, everybody wins.

Personal Growth Well Beyond Adolescence

Psychologically and emotionally, a person's 50s and 60s can be a time of involution and ceasing to create. This is the personal challenge that baby boomers will face in the next two decades. Do they continue creating new ideas and enterprises and contributing in meaningful ways to society, or do they withdraw into a cocoon of isolation, self-involvement, and dependency on others?

During the 1950s, Americans developed a normative expectation that workers would rely on social guarantees to withdraw from work for the last decades of their lives. By doing so, they withdrew not only from their work-related social networks but also from the psychological and economic rewards of continued activity. We now realize that many of them placed their health, physical and emotional, at risk when they did so.

Baby boomers' parents' and grandparents' lives were framed by the terrifying economic collapse of the Great Depression, followed by a remarkable societal renewal of the New Deal and the triumph of World War II. The Depression and war engendered in their survivors both caution and fatalism, as well as a deep faith in the power of government.

Boomers grew up in a period of sustained prosperity, in which they could afford to fail and yet gain new opportunities. Boomers are also as a generation optimistic about their personal futures. It isn't merely evangelical Christians or Buddhists who believe in "rebirth." The United States is a country of new beginnings. Our country's national bird should be not the eagle but rather the phoenix.

Like some of their parents' generation, more than a few baby boomers are already exhausted by life's slings and arrows. But many millions of other boomers will not cease "beginning anew" merely because they have reached their 60s or 70s. For them, these decades will bring a fresh wave of new ideas, new ventures, and new work and voluntary service roles. This fresh wave of creative energy will create new jobs, new products, and, if successful, new tax revenues or other social benefits.

Baby boomers, who have challenged every other social norm they faced, appear poised to diverge from their parents' and grandparents' life trajectories yet again in the next thirty years. Technology and the changing nature of work in the global knowledge economy have reinforced the predisposition of boomers to remain engaged and connected to work, as well as to volunteer their services to their communities. Capitalizing on this energy, and the wealth and knowledge it will create, is the central task of creating a constructive social policy for the baby boom's final act.

Access to health benefits will be a key mediating influence in baby boomers' ability to work longer. Once they reach the age of eligibility for Medicare, however, they will confront a forty-three-year-old federal health program created for a health system fundamentally different (and more primitive) than today's, one designed for a different generation of older Americans. How that program must be modernized, simplified, and refocused to help baby boomers remain healthy longer is the subject of the next chapter.

six

Medicare

The Mount Everest of Entitlements

The fastest-growing social program for older Americans, Medicare, has itself reached midlife. In 2005 the Medicare program turned 40. "Before Medicare" in health care is like "before computing" in the business world. Medicare was enacted in 1965—before open-heart surgery, before biotechnology, before radiation therapy, before arthroscopy and colonoscopy. Film-based X-ray was the principal means of noninvasive diagnosis, and the only definitive way of resolving diagnostic uncertainty was exploratory surgery inside the body cavity or brain. Radical mastectomy was the definitive treatment for breast cancer, and ambulatory surgery, except for the removal of warts and cysts, was essentially unheard of. Pharmaceuticals were defined primarily by the post–World War II regimen of antibiotics.

Medicare was designed to address what were, at the time, the two major health care expenses for older citizens: hospitalization and physician care. Physician care in 1965 not only was inexpensive but also was provided by generalist physicians such as internists and family practitioners. Surgical care was provided in large part by general surgeons. Subspecialty medicine and surgery were in their infancy.

In the ensuing forty years, subspecialties such as cardiology, orthopedic surgery, gastroenterology, and urology—crucial to caring for older patients—have flourished (thanks, in large measure, to Medicare itself). These disciplines have acquired remarkable and expensive diagnostic tools such as flexible fiberoptic scopes and MRI and computed tomographic (CT) scanning, as well as lasers, high-technology implants for joint replacement, and a host of powerful implantable devices. The volume of procedures using these less-invasive technologies, not hospitalization or physician visits, is what today powers Medicare expenses skyward.

This chapter discusses why the Medicare program needs to be fundamentally rethought and restructured and outlines a four-step reform agenda that can both slow the growth of its cost and better focus Medicare on improving the health of baby boomers.

Scaling Mount Everest

Medicare is the Mount Everest of federal entitlement programs. By itself, Medicare is more than half the size of the GDP of Mexico.[1] In fiscal 2005, Medicare spent about $342 billion to provide medical services to those over age 65. In fiscal 2007, this amount jumped to $444.7 billion with the incorporation of a prescription drug benefit.[2] (Even with this large increase, however, Medicare represented only 22% of total U.S. health spending.)

Future Medicare spending is central to the catastropharian nightmare. That is because the present value of Medicare, as well as Medicaid and other future promised health services to the baby boomers and their younger brothers and sisters, has been estimated at approximately $50 trillion of the $72 trillion in present value of future social spending liabilities.[3]

Like most long-range budget estimates, which are reliably unreliable, these forecasts contain many straight-line extrapolations of current trends. They assume historical health status and health care use patterns of older Americans will continue and that existing payment incentives (and their inflationary bias) will remain unchanged long into the future. These Medicare spending forecasts are highly sensitive to assumptions of future cost growth, which seem to change almost annually in ways that materially affect the projected "final" cost.[4]

However dubious the validity of future Medicare cost growth forecasts, the need to modernize this program does not depend on the impending senior boom. *If there were no impending increase in the number of Medicare beneficiaries,* the program as currently designed poses a threat to not only the federal budget but also the U.S. economy as a whole.

Medicare is like a Camaro Z-28, a high-powered fiscal gas-guzzler. Medicare's payment framework is not only fragmented and bewilderingly complex. It is also inherently inflationary as well as biased toward a style of health care increasingly out of phase with the needs of older Americans. Getting better mileage out of Medicare spending, as well as reinforcing a baby boomer inclination toward healthier living, is essential to avoiding the catastropharian nightmare.

Although not by the conscious intent of its designers, Medicare payment policy rewards health care providers for waiting until something is seriously wrong with a beneficiary before intervening, and then lavishes taxpayer dollars on those who do the intervening. Under the present Medicare payment scheme, the program pays principally for "bottom of the cliff " medicine—repairing the damage from long-established disease processes such as heart disease and diabetes only after they threaten the life and independence of older people.

The big money, and therefore the most intense focus, in heart care, for example, is not on the prosaic tasks of controlling hypertension or reducing cholesterol, but on the brinksmanship of cardiac diagnostics and open-heart surgery, late-stage interventions in a preventable, life-threatening crisis that has been decades in the making. By covering prescription drug spending, the Medicare Modernization Act of 2003 went a considerable distance toward rectifying some of the prevention problem (e.g., by covering beta blockers and statins), while failing abjectly to address the skewed incentives rewarding expensive, acute intervention.

Compelling financial incentives to perform expensive tests and procedures have resulted in sustained double-digit growth in the volume of procedures for Medicare beneficiaries and, many observers believe, a lot of expensive care of marginal benefit to patients.[5] Despite recent earnest efforts by Congress to encourage some forms of prevention (such as covering mammograms as well as a "welcome to Medicare" health assessment for newly enrolled beneficiaries), Medicare continues to pay inadequately for primary and preventive care. Primary care practitioners who rely on the Medicare program for most of their income are courting insolvency.[6]

Acute Care Solutions to Chronic Disease Problems

Biological aging is accumulating overlapping chronic illnesses—degenerative diseases of the bones and joints such as arthritis; declining capacity of the liver, kidney, and lungs; failing eyesight and hearing; and degenerative conditions of the brain, beginning with memory loss and culminating in serious, life-threatening symptoms of Parkinson's or Alzheimer's disease. A sufficient accumulation of these deficits prevents older people not only from working but also from living independently.

Accumulating disability also makes older people with these conditions exceptionally vulnerable to accidents or opportunistic illnesses such as pneumonia. Though, as was earlier discussed, disability rates among older Americans are declining at an accelerating rate, chronic illness is still the principal cost burden for the Medicare program. Traditional Medicare paid for attention to chronic care only to the extent that the services were related to recovering from an episode of hospitalization. Even today, Medicare finances "aftercare," not "before care," for chronic disease that represents the bulk of the older person's significant health risks.

Medicare's bias toward acute medicine historically excluded from coverage most forms of chronic care, such as skilled nursing care or home health care, other than when they were directly tied to a hospital discharge. Though there has been some broadening of eligibility for home health care services for conditions not directly linked to hospitalization, most of the cost and inconvenience associated with chronic health problems have been shifted to the families of older people.[7]

Unpaid family caregivers, overwhelmingly women, absorb huge costs not only in anxiety but also in inability to remain employed. An estimated 33.8 million adults participate in this informal care system for family members, contributing an average of almost eighteen hours of unpaid care a week.[8] According to Ken Dychtwald, "the average 21st Century American will actually spend more years caring for parents than for children."[9]

A Bias toward Action

Medicare's coverage and payment policies are not solely to blame for an unaffordable national health care bill. They mirror the core incentives of private health plans. Physicians frequently blame the need for lavish testing and intervention for all their patients, not just older ones, on their malpractice risk—the danger that underdiagnosing or undertreating a medical condition may land them in front of a hostile jury.

There is a germ of truth to this argument: much inappropriate medical expense has been added to our nation's medical expense by our tort liability system.[10] I am an advocate of tort reform and believe it has an important role to play in more affordable health care. But the moral validity of physicians' claims that tort liability drives them to prescribe and treat more aggressively and defensively than appropriate is undercut at least in part by the fact that excessive diagnostic tests and invasive procedures are highly profitable to the physicians who perform them (increasingly the same physicians who order them). The situation is analogous to that of the taxi driver who happily takes the "great circle route" to your destination and tells you that it is safer than going there by a shorter route.

Medicare patients and families also bear responsibility for Medicare's cost escalation. Despite the fact that much disease among older Americans is either self-limiting or "incurable," Medicare has abetted a "bias toward action" by both the health care system and the patient. Like most Americans, Medicare beneficiaries believe that doing *something* about a medical problem is inherently better than waiting. Unlike the privately insured population, however, most Medicare patients are completely sheltered from the final cost of expensive care. Because the marginal cost to Medicare patients of much expensive care is effectively zero, patient pressure on physicians to use expensive clinical services is intensified.

The degree of patient exposure to the cost of care under Medicare is an artifact of forty years of tinkering. There is comparatively large exposure to the cost of a hospitalization, in which the beneficiary is likely to have little influence on the decision, and negligible exposure to the cost of a surgeon's fee for elective surgery or a high-tech imaging procedure, in which there is much greater physician discretion and moral hazard.[11]

There is, on the other hand, enormous exposure (conceivably millions of dollars) to the cost of a serious illness on the "back end," because there is no catastrophic cap on the total cost to the Medicare patient and little patient control over expenses. With the new Medicare prescription drug benefit, all beneficiaries, regardless of their income or medical condition, also face a several-thousand-dollar gap in coverage (the so-called doughnut hole) when their annual drug costs exceed $2,250. After out-of-pocket spending reaches $3,600, the plan pays 95 percent of drug costs.[12]

It has been estimated that the *average* Medicare beneficiary without supplemental insurance will incur almost $190,000 in lifetime costs for cost sharing of Medicare's *covered* services (e.g., not including long-term care costs).[13] As a direct result, more than 85 percent of Medicare beneficiaries are sheltered from any cost exposure to care decisions through supplemental insurance. Of this group, 10 percent have that exposure covered by Medicaid because they have either no assets, low incomes, or both. Another 30 percent have employer-based retiree coverage, 31 percent have supplemental MediGap insurance purchased as individuals, and 15 percent have comprehensive coverage through private health plans (under so-called Part C of Medicare).

Thus, of the 42 million Medicare beneficiaries, fewer than 15 percent have exposure to the cost of the care they receive. By comparison, only 17 percent of the 160 million people with corporate-sponsored health coverage have so-called first-dollar coverage.[14] A far larger percentage of older Americans simply insure away cost exposure under Medicare supplementation rather than enroll in managed care plans. The issue of who shares what costs for what services has not been systematically examined; it has merely accumulated in politically rigid program structures over forty-three years. At present, the vast majority of the economic risk of future Medicare cost increases is borne by younger workers who support the program with their payroll deductions and income taxes.

A High-Maintenance Annuity for Health Care Providers

Because Medicare has formidable economic power with physicians, hospitals, and other health care providers, the federal government has been able to restrain the overall program cost below that of employer-based private health insurance for all but a handful of the past twenty years. It has done this by using its economic leverage as a dominant purchaser of health services to fix both hospital rates and physician fees through a complex system of price controls such as are used in more centralized health care systems in Canada and Europe.

These price controls are a mechanical substitute for a better balancing of the risk of future health care costs among patients, health care providers, and taxpayers. Price controls also have the unfortunate political effect of converting the discussion about how providers are paid into a second type of entitlement—the entitlement of Medicare-dependent providers to an income. Medicare policy has become, in actuality, an "incomes" policy for the vast U.S. health care system. And despite its modest success relative to private health insurance in containing costs, Medicare's spending has still risen at between double and triple the rate of inflation for most of the past twenty years.

Medicare payment and coverage policy is inherently inflationary, because it has masked both the cost and the value of care to the patient, while presenting powerful financial incentives for physicians to call in colleagues to consult on medical problems, to order expensive tests such as MRI scans and panels of laboratory tests, and to intervene aggressively in situations of clinical uncertainty. The more services they perform, the more Medicare pays them.

It is a testimony to the stubborn persistence of ethical standards in medicine that not all U.S. physicians choose to practice this way. Though only a handful of health policy experts seem to care, the annual amount of spending per Medicare beneficiary varies by nearly *threefold* depending on where he or she lives (figure 6.1). In diverse communities such as Bangor, Maine; Grand Rapids, Michigan; Omaha, Nebraska; and Portland, Oregon, physicians practice a far more conservative brand of medicine, passing up opportunities to enrich themselves by caring for Medicare patients.

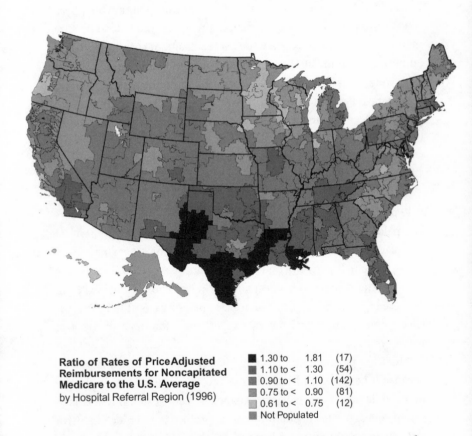

Ratio of Rates of Price Adjusted Reimbursements for Noncapitated Medicare to the U.S. Average by Hospital Referral Region (1996)

■ 1.30 to	1.81	(17)
■ 1.10 to <	1.30	(54)
■ 0.90 to <	1.10	(142)
■ 0.75 to <	0.90	(81)
■ 0.61 to <	0.75	(12)
■ Not Populated		

Figure 6.1. Variation in Medicare Part A/Part B payment, by market area, 1996
Source: Dartmouth Atlas of Health Care, 1999. http://www.dartmouthatlas.org/atlases/atlas_series.shtm.

In other communities, many in the nation's Sunbelt, but also in parts of the Northeast, however, physicians have learned to "mine" older patients, loading them up with specialist consultations and expensive diagnostic tests and performing high-risk procedures often of dubious value. And there is evidence that the increased services do not improve health status, but rather the reverse.[15]

Diffuse Accountability for Patient Care

As it has grown, Medicare has accommodated a practice style in which multiple physicians work on the same patient without communicating with one another or coordinating their activities. In some communities, a hospitalized Medicare patient may have as many as a dozen consulting physicians he or she may never see again. Each is paid separately, and the payment for all physicians is separated from the hospital payment for each admission. This bias toward multiple autonomous actors is, again, not unique to Medicare; it replicates the private financing systems like Blue Cross and Blue Shield on which Medicare payment was modeled when the program was created in 1965. These programs have historically respected the right of each physician to make decisions (and be paid) in complete isolation from others caring for the same patient.

The lack of communication among multiple health care providers, however, has a particularly dangerous side effect for older patients: polypharmacy. A Medicare beneficiary fills, on average, 23 prescriptions per year.[16] Visit an older relative's medicine cabinet sometime, and you will see the problem with your own eyes: dozens of vials of medications prescribed by as many as a half dozen different physicians. You will find expired prescriptions that may no longer be clinically effective. Or you will find prescriptions partly consumed, abandoned before they could do what they were supposed to. Or you will find prescriptions for drugs that were never intended to be taken together due to toxic drug-drug interactions. And because they were prescribed by physicians who did not communicate with one another, no one except the pharmacy that filled them understood the risks.

The Food and Drug Administration, as part of its rigorous drug approval process, requires that each individual drug be exhaustively screened for toxic effects, both in laboratory cell culture and in functioning human beings (most often young, white, and male), before it is approved for broader use. However, the FDA does not perform the real-world test of what happens when the new drug is added to a complex soup of fifteen other medications, taken at odd times and in varying doses by a frail, memory-impaired, eighty-three-year-old woman.

As the older patient's cognitive powers diminish, this arsenal of drugs becomes progressively more dangerous to his or her health. Medication errors account for as many as 30,000 deaths a year in *hospitals*, where a nursing staff and charting system is available to help keep track of the use of the drugs.[17] The number of adverse drug events outside hospitals has not been reliably estimated but may be five to seven times as prevalent.

According to a study in *JAMA*, medication-related injuries among older patients seen in an ambulatory setting are both common and often preventable.[18] If the findings of this study were generalized to the population of 38 million Medicare enrollees, it would suggest that more than 1.9 million adverse drug events occur in this population each year.[19]

The Looming Physician Shortage

As if all these problems were not enough, an antiquated Medicare physician payment system is conspiring with the impending retirement of baby boom physicians to create a crisis of access to physicians' services when baby boomers begin enrolling in Medicare in 2011. Currently, 25 percent of Medicare beneficiaries report difficulty finding a new physician.[20]

This problem will likely worsen with a wave of impending physician retirements. According to the American Medical Association, some 38 percent of practicing physicians in the United States are over the age of 50. Recent surveys suggest that as many as half of physicians plan to make a change in their practices in the next few years. More than a third would like to leave practice, either transitioning into management or retiring outright.[21]

In the next one to three years, more than a quarter of older physicians plan to see only existing patients. Many physicians in the 50–60 age group will seek alternatives to patient care, resulting in millions of patient visits per year from their patients being absorbed by other practicing physicians.[22] The ability of boomer physicians to gear down or retire will be constrained by the adequacy of their pension funding, which was, like that of millions of other Americans, savaged by the technology stock collapse of 2000.

In the eventuality of a sustained rise in stock prices (we are in the fifth year of a stock market rally as of this writing) that renders physicians' retirement from practice affordable, millions of older Americans may find themselves looking for new physicians just as the first wave of baby boomers becomes eligible to enroll in the Medicare program. Depending on the regional medical marketplace, many of these newly entitled boomer Medicare beneficiaries will feel like they have a large red M on their forehead and are likely to have difficulty finding physicians to care for them.

Medicare's budget rules have restricted growth in physician fees since 1999 to attempt to manage the cost of the program. Except in 2001, formula-driven fee reductions have been rolled back by Congress at the last minute, but legal requirements to actually cut physician fees will remain until Medicare physician payment policy can be fundamentally reexamined. Policy debates about how to avoid a physician access crunch under Medicare revolve, predictably, around increasing fees to physicians rather than changing how physicians are paid to encourage better service and better health for Medicare recipients.

The Medicare Policy Stalemate

The main axis of political debate over the future of Medicare for the past fifteen years has been the neoconservative desire to "outsource" Medicare to private health plans, converting Medicare from an open-ended service entitlement to a financing vehicle that would leave the dirty work to private plans. Budgeting under such a system would be reduced to a simple calculation of the appropriate rate of increase in payments by Medicare to private health plans; the "marketplace" would presumably do the rest. Medicare would be out of the price control business. Neoconservative economic dogma holds that private plans can use their presumed market power more effectively than the government to contain the expense of caring for older people. This argument has been mooted to a large extent because much of private health plan market power has disappeared in the past few years due to both hospital mergers and the increasing scarcity of physicians.

After more than two decades of fiddling with the incentives to enroll Medicare beneficiaries in private health care plans, no more than 20 percent of Medicare beneficiaries have chosen to do so despite generous subsidies to the plans to take on the additional risk. Medicare currently pays the plans substantially more than the actual cost of caring for Medicare beneficiaries in the regular program. This seems intuitively like a bad bargain, because the rationale for health plan involvement in Medicare in the first place was to reduce unnecessary care and hold health care providers accountable for cost. It ought to cost less than fee-for-service Medicare, not more, particularly because Medicare beneficiaries who enroll in private plans are healthier than the average Medicare beneficiary. Here, again, however, the politics of Medicare's "incomes policy" for health plans will constrain efforts to rationalize payment.

While they remain an important part of the program, private health care plans are not going to replace traditional Medicare as the dominant source of funding for older Americans in our lifetime. The outsourcing debate has forestalled for more than a decade any serious discussion of the need to renovate the traditional Medicare program itself, which serves almost 35 million older Americans. While policy makers fought over the role of the private plans, the core problem of the flawed incentives and fragmentation inherent in the historical program have remained unaddressed. In addition to explosive growth in Part B premiums, which boomers will pay in part themselves out of their Social Security checks, traditional Medicare's confusing structure and coverage policies will baffle and irritate baby boomers, who are used to receiving coverage from a single source.

Dividing health care payment for services to older Americans into four separate programs makes neither clinical nor economic sense in a twenty-first-century health care system. The division of Medicare into Part A (hospital inpatient) and Part B (physician and outpatient services) dates from the Blue Cross/Blue Shield split of the 1930s and is thus of comparable antiquity to Social Security itself. Payment for most long-term care to older Americans is financed through the Medicaid program, administered separately by the fifty states. Recent reform efforts further increased the complexity of the program. The so-called Medicare Modernization Act of 2003 added yet a fourth part, Part D for drugs, further fragmenting payment. (Part C is the private health plan enrollment option.) Part D coverage is provided only through private health plans.

How Medicare pays hospitals, doctors, and others for caring for older Americans has also not kept pace with a changing world. After a burst of innovation in the 1980s and early 1990s, Medicare payment policy has stagnated in the past decade. Though Medicare has begun cautiously experimenting with pay-for-performance for health care providers, Medicare hospital payment policy remains frozen in the 1980s, while its fee-for-service physician payment model represents an only modestly updated version of the method used to pay Hippocrates in ancient Greece almost 2,500 years ago, overlaid with a stunning and steadily increasing level of technical and operational complexity.

Reform is by no means neither technically nor politically impossible. Medicare made history in the early 1980s by changing its hospital payment strategy from paying à la carte for each day of care and each service provided to paying hospitals on a prix-fixe per-admission basis (using diagnosis-related groups, or DRGs). This seemingly trivial change had a major impact on restraining program cost, and encouraged hospitals and physicians to work together in caring for Medicare patients by rewarding them for shortening Medicare beneficiaries' hospital stays and economizing on tests and medications. Hospital use plummeted in the ensuing several years, while patients barely noticed the difference.[23]

Less-publicized changes in Medicare's physician compensation and outpatient hospital payment strategy in the 1990s attempted to correct payment inequities between primary care physicians and specialists and encourage economies in outpatient care, but had negligible effect on physician behavior or quality of service.

Starting Over?

Peter Drucker once famously advised corporate leaders to ask themselves if they would be in the business they are currently in if they had to start fresh. If you were designing the Medicare program afresh for today's technologies and tomorrow's seniors (baby boomers), you wouldn't build the Medicare program we have today.

If you were starting afresh, you would not separate Medicare benefits into large, rigid categories (hospital inpatient, physician and ambulatory services, prescription drugs, and long-term care services are the four big ones), as the present program does. You would also not pay health care providers, in effect, not to cooperate with one another or to maximize the volume of services they offer. Rather than having multiple, or a dozen, physicians responsible for separate medical conditions, you would encourage beneficiaries to choose a single point of contact for the health care system who could see the entire picture of a person's health, including medications.

Medicare beneficiaries would choose a "single point of contact" physician, based on their medical needs and past relationships, and that physician would receive a monthly fee from Medicare for maintaining the relationship, covering visits and electronic and telephone contacts with the patient, as well as preventive care. You would reward health-promoting relationships between this central health care provider and the patient, and pay for maintaining those relationships on a "subscription" basis, rather than rewarding the number of expensive tests, procedures, and patient visits those providers generate.

When you turn on the relationship, it's "always on," and information can flow from the health care system to the person and back more or less continuously. Medicare would insist on and pay for evidence-based medical practice and would reward with higher payments those who do a better job of keeping their patients healthy. Providers who agreed to use scientifically validated clinical pathways, use chronic-care disease-management programs, and encourage their patients to manage their clinical risks more effectively would be paid on a simpler and more generous basis than the present fee-for-service system does.

Medicare would aggressively promote clinical information technology to reduce medical errors, duplicative testing, and inappropriate diagnoses. You would insist that health care providers all use a single common, electronic record for each patient to manage the care provided, so that everyone who touches the patient starts from a common and comprehensive knowledge base. You would encourage providers to connect to their high-risk patients through remote clinical monitoring systems that alert them and the families of their subscribers to potential health threats.

Medicare would reward primary care physicians for intervening earlier to prevent illness, using a combination of commonsense behavior modification and high-technology medicines (such as statins and beta-blockers). When someone used an expensive diagnostic tool, such as MRI scanning, or was hospitalized, the patient would pay a meaningful portion of the cost, based on the ability to pay. When someone becomes seriously ill or is injured, rather than paying a dozen different health care providers and the hospital separately, Medicare would make a single unified payment based on the seriousness of the condition and the fragility of the patient, and let the health care system sort out what is needed and how it is provided.

Transactions between Medicare and health care providers and between claims management and payment would be both electronic and instantaneous. Also, there would be far fewer transactions, eliminating much of the vast patient accounts bureaucracy of the nation's hospitals and enabling nurses in physician offices to return to supporting patient care.

Some private health plans that enroll Medicare beneficiaries actually do much of this today. But the hard questions revolve around how to create a more effective, better-focused, easier-to-use benefit for the rest of Medicare's beneficiaries from the confusing and politically gridlocked legacy program we have today. The next four sections of this chapter suggest a stepwise approach to modernizing the Medicare program to prepare for the baby boom.

Fixing Medicare
Step I: Simplify the Traditional Benefit

Today's Medicare beneficiary under the traditional fee-for-service program typically has three separate types of coverage: Medicare coverage itself (Parts A and B), a private MediGap supplement to fill the large financial gaps in the traditional plan, and a private Part D plan to cover drugs. In addition to these three coverages, millions of older Americans have yet a fourth coverage: long-term care insurance to cover the chronic care expenses not covered by Medicare. Those without assets have their long-term care covered by Medicaid.

Baby boomers are going to rebel against the cumbersomeness of these multiple funding mechanisms and the blizzard of paperwork needed to track and pay for the services they need. You need an advanced accounting degree, good record keeping and/or software, and a lot of time to spend on hold listening to Mantovani to actually use the traditional Medicare benefit. It is not, to put it gently, a user-friendly program for an older person with memory impairment or organizational issues.

Currently, the only option that allows the Medicare beneficiary to receive benefits from all four silos (hospital, ambulatory/physician, drug, and long-term care) from a single source is to enroll in a private health plan under Part C of Medicare. As of this writing, about 80 percent of Medicare beneficiaries or their loved ones engage in a confusing involuntary pastime of managing their public benefit from all these diverse sources. (Many of the "lower administrative expenses" that Medicare advocates brag about, relative to private health plans, are actually shifted to patients, their families, and their physicians and hospitals.)

Many people who elect private health plan coverage under Medicare receive superb care. In addition to a more coordinated approach, many private health plans eliminate the billing hassles

Medicare beneficiaries face in a complex illness. For this reason alone, preserving the option for Medicare beneficiaries of enrolling in private health plans makes sense for the oncoming baby boom Medicare users, many of whom have enrolled in managed care plans for most of their working lives and are satisfied with their coverage. The likelihood of getting all Medicare beneficiaries to choose private plans, however, approaches zero. Because the cost to the Medicare program of sponsoring private health plan coverage is presently higher than the cost of fee-for-service Medicare (with wide variation depending on where one lives), it seems unlikely that, even with generous enrollment incentives and a more sophisticated and health-plan-savvy baby boomer population entering Medicare, we will get more than a third of the future Medicare population to choose private plans. For this reason, it is especially important that the traditional Medicare benefit must be dramatically simpler and easier to understand and use.

Recently, health policy specialists at the Urban Institute and Commonwealth Fund proposed a comprehensive redesign for traditional Medicare that not only mirrors the comprehensiveness of the private plans but also, by restructuring patient cost sharing, eliminates the need for most supplemental Medicare insurance. Karen Davis and Marilyn Moon termed this Medicare Extra, or Part E.[24] Part E would also provide a unified benefits package that makes it unnecessary to obtain separate Part D drug coverage and that covers some chronic care services currently not covered by traditional Medicare.

In Davis and Moon's proposal, the patient would pay a $250 deductible, 10 percent copayment for ambulatory and physicians' services, and 25 percent of drug costs. By capping the beneficiary's total out-of-pocket outlays at $3,000, a Part E package would eliminate not only the need for MediGap supplemental insurance but also the hated "doughnut hole" in drug coverage, the least popular feature of the new Medicare drug benefit.

For "Struggling and Anxious" baby boomers, such as Avril Sanchez, who do not have the cash or savings to pay the out-of-pocket expenses, Davis and Moon suggest Medicaid (state government) supplementation based on ability to pay, or a federal supplemental program for low-income people. Alternatively, private health insurers could be encouraged to offer competing supplemental coverage alternatives for lower-income subscribers. Because the gross amount of economic exposure to the cost of care would be lower, the premiums should be much more affordable for those with low incomes or assets. The number of Medicare beneficiaries requiring supplemental help would be dramatically reduced.

By simplifying Medicare's benefit structure and restructuring the patient's cost exposure to focus it better on where patient involvement can control costs (prescription drugs and ambulatory care), the Davis and Moon proposal is a sensible starting point for Medicare reform. It addresses the haphazard and excessive cost exposure of patients by eliminating the need for most beneficiaries to purchase private MediGap coverage. One small and sensible change in their proposal would make the financing system more progressive, by charging higher-income beneficiaries a higher deductible for physician and ambulatory services and by maintaining a somewhat higher annual expense cap for wealthier beneficiaries.

Step II: Change the Incentives to Health Care Providers

Unless payment to hospitals and physicians is modified to encourage better communication and accountability in the health care system, Medicare beneficiaries will not realize the most important benefit of a simplified program—better-coordinated, science-based medical care. Davis and Moon leave in place the existing "administered price" method of paying hospitals, physicians, and other health care providers on an "à la carte," piecework basis.

To achieve better outcomes and affordability, this inflationary, "every man for himself" payment system must be replaced with a better-organized approach.[25] The best way to do this is for Medicare to pay for primary care in what has been called a "medical home." This concept originated in pediatrics to describe a way of organizing care for disabled children, but it has comparable saliency for addressing the health needs of older Americans.[26]

When a Medicare beneficiary enrolls in Part E, he or she should be asked to choose a "medical home"—a single point of contact with the health care system. This single point of contact may be a primary care physician—an internist, family practitioner, or geriatrician—or a community clinic or group practice. The "medical home" will be the home of the patient's electronic health record and the destination of any clinical records from any other clinical encounters with the patient, including prescriptions, hospitalizations, emergency room visits, and consultation by medical or surgical specialists as well as with human services professionals.

In exchange for a single monthly "subscription" payment by Medicare covering office visits, telephone and electronic consultation, patient education, and disease management for those with chronic conditions such as diabetes, asthma, and congestive heart failure, Medicare beneficiaries would be provided with a continuous, 24/7 relationship with the "medical home." Because these services will be covered by a single monthly payment made (electronically) by Medicare, it would not be necessary for beneficiaries to file medical claims for each instance of service, markedly reducing office overhead and administrative costs for their caregivers. Payment levels should be more generous than those associated with the present Part B fee payments for comparable patient populations. Medicare should pay primary care physicians a "living wage" for functioning as a medical home.

The payments to the "medical home" care provider would be "severity adjusted" so that those providers who accepted older or sicker patients receive higher payments to recognize their patients' greater needs. And those who did a more effective job of avoiding hospitalization or clinical complications from diseases identified at the point of enrollment would receive bonus payments to recognize the higher quality of their services. Attaching pay-for-performance bonuses to subscription payments is a more intelligent and less administratively cumbersome way of rewarding performance than tacking it onto medical fees paid for each instance of service (in exchange for a huge increase in administrative cost).

Doing this in the real world is not uncomplicated. During the 1980s, health plans attempted to impose a primitive variant of this model on physicians through something called a "primary care gatekeeper."

Things went horribly awry when health plans insisted that the gate-keeper assume the cost burden of the patient's entire health care and positioned the gatekeeper as the economic adversary of all the other physicians who touched the patient. "Medical home" means not "budget holder" but rather someone with comprehensive knowledge of all the patient's clinical activity and the medications and therapies that result.

When the patient is diagnosed with a clinical condition requiring complex treatment (e.g., congestive heart failure, cancer, or trauma), rather than paying the hospital per admission and each specialist who touches the patient a separate fee, a determination would be made of the clinical condition that required care, as well as the patient's age and comorbid conditions (other illnesses affecting treatment). Then, the enterprise that takes responsibility for the care would receive a single, severity-adjusted payment to cover all services provided to resolve the patient's medical problem, including not only hospitalization and surgery but also any posthospital or rehabilitative care. Because of the single payment, separate medical billings for each service by the hospital and multiple physicians would be unnecessary. Administrative complexity could be reduced markedly for both the health care providers and the patient, and physicians and hospitals could reduce their "back office" billing staffs.

If the organization accepting payment (a hospital system, group practice, or physician or hospital organization) can manage the costs of care for less than the fixed payment (termed by payment wonks a "severity-adjusted case rate"), it can keep the difference (as under present DRG payments to hospitals). If the costs of treating the condition exceed the amount, it absorbs the cost. Because most such enterprises would have thousands of Medicare beneficiaries, the gains and losses are averaged over a large patient population.

This shifting of economic and clinical risk to an organized system of care will encourage not only aggressive use of ambulatory services, avoidance of hospitalization or shorter stays, and substitution of drug treatment for acute intervention, but also aggressive prevention and disease management to avoid repeat hospitalizations or recurrence of the disease.

For health services that fall in the middle, between the "medical home" and the "episode of illness," Medicare beneficiaries would pay Davis and Moon's 10 percent copayment on ambulatory and outpatient services and 25 percent of drug costs, and their providers would be paid as under traditional Medicare—per service they provide. Some thought should be given to higher patient cost sharing (20–30%) for some high-cost and easily abused diagnostic services, such as high-technology imaging (CT and MRI), laboratory testing, and ambulatory surgery, with the cost graded to the income of the beneficiary to avoid income-related inequities in access. Copayments should be waived for preventive care such as periodic mammography, cancer screening, or colonoscopy, to lower cost barriers to preventive care.

A decade ago, only a handful of health care enterprises in the country were sufficiently organized to manage complex care in this way, and even those lacked the clinical information tools to track costs and clinical effectiveness. Many health care providers who tried to do this under so-called capitation payment lost money. Today, however, hundreds of health care enterprises, including teaching hospitals, regional health care systems, integrated group practices, and other organizations, have both the information tools and the relationships with physicians needed to achieve this higher level of organized, science-based care. These enterprises could be expected to step forward and offer both "medical homes" and "accountable health enterprises" to Medicare beneficiaries in their areas that elect a Part E option.

If a large enough number of baby boomers elected this type of benefit, we could expect not only fundamentally superior quality of care for them but also less-explosive growth of cost in Medicare itself. Sensible cost constraints must involve changing incentives and behavior of health care providers and patients together—expecting the patient alone or providers alone to do this is unrealistic and inequitable. Growth in Part E enrollment would also create economic pressure on the remaining fee-for-service Medicare system to reduce unnecessary expenses. Restraining fee increases and hospital expenses under Parts A and B of Medicare would be easier for Congress and the federal government to justify for the providers and patients who chose to remain with a completely open-ended Medicare system.

Step III: Enable People to Buy into Medicare at Age 55

Earlier, I argued that the single greatest barrier to baby boomers following their inclination to work longer is the availability of affordable health coverage. Many boomers are "job locked" because moving to free agency, consultation, or part-time employment deprives them of affordable health benefits. Another problem is that about 4.2 million of the medically uninsured in the United States are between the ages of 55 and 64.[27] While a relatively small group, their health care cost exposure is far higher than that of the more numerous younger uninsured population.

Also, chronic diseases such as heart disease and diabetes become increasingly serious threats to the health of people in the decade before enrollment in Medicare. There is evidence that people in this age band avoid managing those conditions because they lack health coverage, and have persistently higher health costs after enrollment in Medicare (for as long as seven years). The authors of a recent article concluded that "previously uninsured adults used health services more intensively and required costlier care as Medicare beneficiaries than they would have if previously insured." This suggests that traditional Medicare costs could be lowered if people could obtain coverage for chronic conditions earlier.[28]

Enabling people to enroll voluntarily in Medicare at age 55 would not only reduce the number of uninsured Americans but also improve the mobility and employment potential of older workers. This approach is consistent with geriatric expert Christine Cassel's recommendation that the age of eligibility for Medicare be lower than 65 and the age of eligibility for Social Security be higher.[29] The difference here is that early enrollment in Medicare would be voluntary, rather than universal.

Depending on the premiums Medicare charged, underwriting their employed and covered retiree populations' entry into Medicare after age 55 may be a less-expensive option for employers than cover-

ing them through private health insurance. For lower-income or unemployed people older than 55 (e.g., the "Struggling and Anxious"
baby boomers, such as Avril Sanchez), federal subsidy would probably be required. Enrollment premiums and cost sharing ought to
vary based on the ability to pay and be set so that the premium payments are "cost neutral" to the Medicare program (i.e., premiums
paid for 55- to 64-year-olds would cover their anticipated medical
costs).

If this were done, only the subsidies to low-income "early" Medicare
enrollees would represent an additional cost to the program, a cost
that could be justified if, as Ayanian and his colleagues suggest, earlier intervention in preventable illnesses, such as heart disease and
diabetes, could postpone the need for complex medical care.[30] Because sicker potential beneficiaries would be more likely to enroll in
Medicare early, special efforts should be made to incorporate disease
management into their care. Rather than avoiding adverse selection
(e.g., enrolling a disproportionate number of sick people), Medicare
would actively encourage it and anticipate the cost risks by improved
program design.

Broadening the base of Medicare enrollment would give the
Medicare program more clout in increasingly consolidated hospital
markets and discourage physicians, in particular, from dropping
Medicare beneficiaries from their practices. It would also encourage
private health plans to reorganize and strengthen both their cost
management and their customer service to retain their existing enrollments, and to make coverage for older workers more affordable to
business.

Step IV: Allow Working Baby Boomers to Defer Enrollment

If this book's forecast of a healthier baby boomer population is
borne out, and participation in the labor force rises, many of the
working boomers will not need to enroll in Medicare when they
reach age 65 because they will still be insurable by the private sector.
Furthermore, many will have long-standing and satisfactory relationships with managed care health plans or consumer-directed plans.

Present Medicare policy subordinates Medicare coverage to the older worker's private health plan, while compelling beneficiaries to pay Medicare payroll taxes and premiums for services they are not able to use. This seems unjust. Also taxes on Social Security benefits paid to older working beneficiaries are, in part, credited to help pay for some Medicare expenses that workers after age 65 do not incur because their employer's health plan is the primary payer. This also seems unjust.

Why not enable older workers to defer enrollment in Medicare and permit their employers to offset the cost of their health insurance by applying Medicare Part A payroll deductions to help defray their private insurance costs? The incentive for individuals to defer enrollment in Medicare could be a less-costly premium payment when they do enroll. The subsidy for employers to retain their workers older than 65 in privately financed plans could be restricted to health plans that offer health-improvement features such as disease management. As with the earlier suggestion of making Medicare coverage primary for older workers, this would increase Medicare's costs somewhat by diverting payroll taxes currently destined for the Medicare Trust Fund.

Whether this option will be attractive to employers will depend in major part on the cost to them of the previous recommendation. If it costs half as much to subsidize the worker's enrollment in Medicare, few employers will find it advantageous to keep their older workers in their private health plans. The combined effect of these last two policy changes would be to "fuzzify" the use of age of 65 as the threshold to obtaining public health benefits while preserving the universal character of the program.

Addressing the Physician Shortage

Earlier I suggested that older physicians are likely to exit practice coincident with the baby boom's reaching eligibility for Medicare. Averting the impending crisis of access to physician services for Medicare beneficiaries, which will be particularly acute in rural areas, will require aggressive action in federal physician work force policy.

A particular concern is the lack of geriatric specialists. This medical discipline is specially geared to performing the care coordination and management function discussed previously. There are only about 9,000 geriatricians in the United States (compared to 42,000 pediatricians),[31] far fewer than would be needed if the reforms suggested here were implemented.

To fill this gap, the federal government should offer training grants to medical schools to staff their faculties and teaching hospitals to train more geriatricians. Currently, only 5 of the nation's 145 medical schools have departments of geriatric medicine.[32] To encourage greater enrollment, medical students who elect this discipline and pursue it into clinical practice should receive special federal assistance to pay off their medical school loan balances (often more than $200,000) if they stay in geriatric practice six or more years.

Medical schools should also collaborate with their principal teaching hospitals to offer opportunities for internists or family practitioners, or even specialists, for that matter, who wish to make a change in their clinical practice to return to medical education part time and retrain in geriatric medicine. Modern concepts of geriatric care management and many specific disease-management protocols and technologies have developed since older physicians left their training. Programs could also be developed to retrain medical and surgical subspecialists who desire to change their clinical practice to train in primary care medical care disciplines in midcareer. Changing how primary care physicians' services are paid by Medicare, as has been suggested here, will encourage more young people to choose a career in primary care.

There will be intense political pressure both in state legislatures and in Congress to expand medical school enrollments in the next decade as physician access problems worsen. Thought must be given to other strategies for tilting the mix of specialists and primary care physicians back toward primary care as this expansion ensues, to avoid replicating the existing maldistribution of clinical expertise in the face of the eventual rise in medical needs of the baby boom generation. None of these supply side changes will make any difference, however, unless primary medical practice for older Americans pays substantially better than it does today.

Disease-Management Programs

Many of the diseases that affect older Americans have identifiable and controllable risk factors that can be managed by those who have them, to avert or postpone hospitalization or complex therapy. Disease management is "top of the cliff" medicine—approaches that use a combination of medications, assisted behavior change, rich consumer health information, and encouragement to help people manage the early stages of chronic diseases such as asthma, diabetes, hypertension, and even congestive heart failure, which can not only kill subscribers but also generate huge medical bills. A variety of active health-management tools, including intelligent voice-response technology, remote clinical monitoring, and nurse call services, can be integrated and tailored to identifiable clinical risks of patients.

Disease management has special saliency for older subscribers, who are more likely than younger people to struggle with multiple chronic conditions. Disease-management programs for older Americans with congestive heart failure and diabetes have shown the consistent ability to reduce hospitalization rates for these patients, a major driver of Medicare costs.[33] Rather than allowing older Americans to be passive spectators to their own medical risks, disease management is a way to foster their active engagement in addressing and managing those risks before they flower into illness. The Medicare Modernization Act of 2003 sponsored experiments in applying disease-management and care-coordination strategies to Medicare beneficiaries. The goal is to see if disease management can demonstrate results for Medicare beneficiaries that may lead to changes in how Medicare pays for its services.

Many private health plans today offer sophisticated disease-management programs to help subscribers use medications such as beta-blockers to control hypertension, to control their blood sugar more effectively for diabetics, to make sure that women at risk for breast cancer get mammograms, to help people stop smoking or to lose weight—strategies that would not have been welcome in the old "big brother" model of managed care but that fit the "consumer-directed" plan model. These tools need to be adapted to the Medicare population in coming years.

Sacred Cows and Medicare Policy

The universality of coverage at age 65 and an entitlement to defined benefits, as well as Medicare payment policy, are immensely contentious political and social issues. In fact, the economic and political force field surrounding Medicare was so daunting that when the Clintons approached health care reform in 1993, they made what seemed at the time to be a sensible tactical decision to leave the existing Medicare alone (except for adding a drug benefit) and focused on reorganizing private insurance coverage to cover the large population of younger Americans with no health insurance.

This risk aversion may be sensible tactically but questionable strategically. The Medicare program is a potentially crucial actor not only in moderating overall health care cost increases but also in improving the health of Medicare beneficiaries. The traditional role of the Medicare program was simply to passively pay the medical bills accumulated by its beneficiaries. This is not a tenable definition of the program's role going forward.

While the age of enrollment, the structure of the Medicare benefits, and payment incentives are not insignificant issues, they are not as important as the shape of the social contract between baby boomers and society over their health coverage. To produce an affordable outcome, the debate over the future of Medicare needs to be reframed to focus on bringing about an active, engaged Medicare beneficiary.

Baby boomers, particularly women, were the core constituents of the backlash against managed care. They emphatically challenged the managed care plan's right to decide what they needed and when. Boomers have been aggressive users of the health care system. They have also used the Internet to reduce the sharp knowledge gradient between them and their health care providers. They have embraced prevention, as evidenced by the explosive growth in colonoscopy and mammography. For better or worse, baby boomers have tended to want a partnership with health care providers, rather than a parent-child relationship, and want to make informed decisions about their own health with the physician acting as an adviser.

Baby boomers detest paternalism, regardless of who "Dad" is. Boomers do not embrace a paternalist vision of the state's role in their lives. They also do not have the same entitlement mentality as their grandparents and great grandparents, the original grateful beneficiaries of Social Security and Medicare. Unlike the impoverished and poorly educated seniors of the 1960s, contemporary boomers are far better informed about their health risks and many of them are far better endowed economically to pay more of the cost of the care. That wealth and knowledge is unequally distributed, however, challenging those who craft social policy to assure both just and fair distribution of public benefits and to assure that the most vulnerable among the baby boomers are protected.

It is important to protect all Americans from the inevitable and expensive landing at the bottom of the cliff and to spread the cost of "bottom of the cliff " care over as broad a population base as possible. For this reason, Medicare needs to remain universal. Eventually, we will all be on Medicare. But we also need to expend much greater energy and creativity to helping Medicare beneficiaries avoid landing at the bottom of the cliff for as long as humanly possible and to implicate older Americans, *both morally and economically,* in making the personal decisions to avoid or postpone illness.

Health care providers need to participate in the sharing of responsibility. They should do so by how they are paid; profit should not inhere in delivering more care to Medicare recipients whether it is needed or not. If there is profit, it should derive from maintaining healthy relationships with patients and practicing conservative, evidence-based medical care. Tampering with the health system's food supply is dangerous politically but unavoidable if these changes are to occur.

As was suggested earlier, Medicare is like Mount Everest in the U.S. political system, and, like Mount Everest, it makes its own weather. Incautious politicians who wish to scale it and plant their flag can find themselves freezing to death in a howling wind near the summit. Powerful political and social forces sustain the risk-free flow of Medicare funding to hospitals, physicians, and technology companies and resist any diminution of provider income or professional prerogatives.

The breadth and shape of the Medicare program goes directly to what it means to be a citizen. The social contract between baby boomers and the Medicare program should assume that Medicare beneficiaries are knowledgeable grown-ups who can influence both their own health and the ultimate cost of the care they receive by making intelligent decisions in collaboration with their physicians and family members. Encouraging older Americans to become actively engaged in managing their own health is the key to an affordable, healthier older population. Baby boomers are not going to behave like their grandparents did forty years ago; to foster their active engagement in improving their health is not an imposition; it fits their personal values and goals. It is also the only socially responsible alternative to the present passive entitlement to care whose costs loom over the mid-twenty-first century.

As I discuss further in chapter 7 on Social Security, public benefits and private benefits must mesh better and give older workers the flexibility to determine how these benefits are deployed, given their unique needs. "One size fits all" is neither an affordable nor a practical approach to structuring public benefits to older Americans. Without changes that simplify the Medicare benefit, Medicare risks the rapid loss of baby boomer political support as larger numbers of them become eligible and enroll.

seven

Social Security Reform

Grasping the Third Rail

The future promises of Social Security are dwarfed by those of the Medicare program, but according to Kotlikoff's economic model, they still amount to more than $22 trillion, or almost double our current GDP.[1] Social Security lacks the focused attention of a $2.1 trillion health industry and its well-paid "public defenders." This does not seem to have made reforming Social Security any easier. Baby boomers, who believe they are much younger than their chronological age, are looking backward at their youth, not forward toward the easy chair. Most of my boomer colleagues have not spent even ten minutes thinking about how Social Security is going to affect them.

As with Medicare, however, boomers will in the next few years encounter a Social Security program designed for an industrial economy and for their fragile great grandparents. Even if many economists (and the financial services industry) believe that baby boomers and their younger brothers and sisters are "underreserved" for retirement, whenever it occurs, how the Social Security system should help fill this gap has occasioned the bitterest domestic political debate in the past decade. This political debate has been both depressingly polarized and extravagantly unproductive.

George Bush's Domestic Policy Bungee Jump

When George W. Bush returned to Washington in early 2005 to begin his ill-starred second term, he announced his intention, as he put it, to invest his political capital in renovating the Social Security system. His initiative startled many in the policy and political community. Social Security reform was not a centerpiece of his reelection campaign, which focused on the Global War on Terror. Nor did Social Security address his core constituency of economic and evangelical conservatives, except in the tangential sense of potentially creating more mutual fund investors.

By taking on Social Security reform, Bush hurled himself and his political capital at one of the most emotionally fraught creations of twentieth-century U.S. politics, the centerpiece of Franklin Roosevelt's New Deal. Conventional political wisdom suggested that Social Security was the "third rail" of American politics: touch it and die.

The centerpiece of Bush's Social Security reform proposal was to create voluntary, privately held accounts to be owned and managed by the beneficiary. These private accounts would have been funds that Congress could not spend because it could not reach them. Bush's proposal was funded by redirecting some of the system's current cash flow—4 percentage points of workers' payroll tax deductions up to $1,000 a year—into private accounts.[2] The theory was that if voluntary private accounts under Social Security were invested in equities or bonds, they could earn more than if invested in government securities, as the program currently does.

Bush's reform proposals were targeted at politically disengaged Gen X and Gen Y voters (who voted overwhelmingly for Bush's Democratic opponent in 2004). Only 31 percent of these young people believe Social Security will be available for them upon retirement.[3] Most young people know little about Social Security and seemingly could care less. Not surprisingly, their silence on the subject of Social Security reform has been deafening.

Older Americans, on the other hand, have been traditionally *very* anxious about any change in Social Security. This is for the excellent reason that two-thirds of them depend on it for as much as half of their total income. Some 25 percent depend exclusively on it for their livelihoods.[4] Bush was quick to assure these important people that there would be no change in their monthly check.

In the broad populace, baby boomers split almost fifty-fifty on the need for private accounts, with a slight majority opposing Bush's specific proposals. AARP surveys, however, have shown that a significant majority of baby boomers are willing to support some type of Social Security reform, including the creation of private investment accounts.[5] So Bush's proposal failed to actuate the latent support among boomers for change in the program. With the deafening silence from younger people and adamant opposition from current retirees and their advocates (despite Bush's reassurances that their checks will be unimpaired), Social Security reform went precisely nowhere.

Bush's proposals were brushed aside by Congress. This was not only because Bush was twisting in the hot winds of the Iraq war, but also because Democrats did not feel enough political pressure to offer counterproposals. However, the reason Social Security reform has gone nowhere is because, for the vast majority of baby boomers (the core of the American electorate), Bush's proposals offered nothing except uncertainty. The majority of representatives in Congress regard Social Security reform as a *very* risky political agenda item. Many also happen to be baby boomers themselves and can easily calculate the political risks and consequences of this uncertainty.

Crisis Not Imminent but Readily Apparent

Despite the rhetoric of imminent crisis, Social Security's day of reckoning is, in fact, about a decade away. Social Security's present role in the federal government is that of cash cow: every year it takes in more than $150 billion more than it disperses to older, widowed, or disabled people. Some younger people—and even a few baby boomers, for that matter—who do not pay close attention to the arcana of Social Security's accounting think this cash is going into a Trust Fund that is both physically segregated and invested wisely to protect benefit payouts for them when they are needed.

Of course, those who have been paying attention know that this is not the case. Into the Social Security Trust Fund goes not cash to be sheltered for later use, but government bonds that must be cashed out at some future date to pay benefits. The Trust Fund cookie jar contains not real cookies but IOUs—more than $1.8 trillion in interest-bearing U.S. government securities, which are promises to buy cookies with current cash in some future year.[6] (The interest is also paid in IOUs.)

Under a "pay-as-you-go" approach, Social Security needed only to collect enough cash to fund current year outlays to this year's retirees (and survivors and disabled people) from the paychecks of younger workers. The excess in Social Security taxes over those current pay-outs (which was generated by a huge 1983 tax increase designed to "permanently" cure the system's long-term financial imbalance) has been treated as "free money" to be spent according to the whims and pressures of the political moment. Thus, the surplus Social Security cash is actually being spent on the war in Iraq, Homeland Security, subsidies to tobacco growers, rainforests in Iowa, and other pressing current needs. During his ill-fated presidential campaign in 2000, Al Gore made a much-parodied proposal to sequester Social Security's surplus cash flow in a "lock box" so Congress could not squander it. It was difficult to generate electoral outrage about this process not only because voters did not understand it but also because there was no federal budget deficit at the time.

Social Security's big problem comes in 2017. In that year, cash coming in from workers' payroll deductions is expected to be out-stripped by benefit payments to that year's beneficiaries. After 2017, Social Security goes, as they say in the corporate world, "cash flow negative." To pay its obligations to Social Security beneficiaries in that year, the federal government will need to find $23 billion in cash to meet its obligations, an amount that grows to *$400 billion* a year in 2028.[7]

To meet those cash needs, the federal government will have to sell (to itself) the treasury securities in the Trust Fund. The Trust Fund will be completely empty of IOUs by 2042. For Social Security's fun-damentalists to claim that there is no problem until 2042 is utter hogwash. While U.S. treasury securities are as reliable as there is in the world of debt instruments, they must still be redeemed *in cash* for Social Security to pay its bills. The cash has to come from somewhere. It will have to come from the federal treasury and, therefore, the pockets of future taxpayers.

If the economy happens, by happy coincidence, to be growing in 2017, solving the Social Security funding problem will merely require allocating some of the billions in new federal tax revenues from prosperity to begin redeeming the Trust Fund's IOUs. If the economy is in trouble, there will be a lot of claimants on federal funding (poor people, city governments, national parks, the navy, etc.), who could find themselves sent to the back of the line so that newly entitled (if not actually retired) baby boomers can have their promised benefits.

Despite the fact that Bush's proposed private accounts offset some future Social Security payments to those who created them, Bush's proposal deepened the system's eventual need for cash and moved up the "cash negative" date from 2017. This is because current payroll deductions funneled into private investment accounts "owned" by younger workers could not be paid out to current retirees.

Crisis of Legitimacy

Social Security's problems run deeper, however, than a shortfall of promised funding. The social compact between people and their government, of which Social Security was a key component, is fraying around the edges. Faith in the legitimacy of government's role in people's lives is in short supply. In a 2007 Democracy Corps poll, 57 percent of likely voters agreed with the statement "government makes it harder for people to get ahead in life" compared with 29 percent who believed that "government does more to help people get ahead in life." Those in the prime earning years from ages 30 to 50 had even higher levels of disillusionment. Of those polled, 63 percent disapproved of government performance on Social Security and 80 percent on government spending in general.[8]

This absence of trust goes directly to the viability of government as an agent of social solidarity, an original motivation of the framers of

Social Security. If the people doing the subsidizing—that is, the working population—do not trust the federal government, they will not support changes in Social Security that promote its solvency. For the very reason that Congress could not reach and squander the sequestered funds, the augmentation of Social Security with voluntary private accounts could help strengthen the program's legitimacy, provided that they could be funded responsibly.

Who "Owns" Social Security's Assets?

Disentangling the intergenerational subsidy flows is also essential, however, if restive generations of younger voters are not eventually to support gutting the program. Current beneficiaries believe that what they receive in benefits actually belongs to them—that they have been paying insurance premiums for a publicly guaranteed annuity all their working lives. Under the logic of social insurance, the system is simply returning to them, with some ill-defined return on their capital, what they put in. Current workers also believe they "own" the funding they contribute in each paycheck to Social Security. Generations of well-meaning political leaders have led both current workers and current retirees to believe that what they contribute or receive back from the program belongs to them.

This is not what is actually happening. The reality is that the newly enrolled Social Security beneficiary gets back his or her contributions, plus a minuscule return (e.g., the interest on the government securities, which in the 1950s and part of the 1960s was less than 2% per year), *plus* a hefty subsidy from current workers, who simultaneously believe that their payroll contributions are funding a future benefit that belongs only to them. Because all of a beneficiary's cash contributions have already been spent, every penny of the cash that beneficiaries receive in their Social Security checks actually comes from *current* wage earners.

Depending on their lifetime earnings, two-income retired couples who become eligible for Social Security and Medicare benefits in 2010 will receive between 11 percent and 47 percent more than what they put into Social Security and as much as 3.3 to 6.7 times as much as what they put in to Medicare.[9] The difference is a net subsidy from younger workers and taxpayers. These subsidies will increase as health care costs rise in the future and will rise most dramatically for the sickest Medicare beneficiaries who use the most services. Many in the social policy community have traditionally viewed this double counting as a magical compact that binds young and old together. But only in a magical world can both generations successfully own the same dollar.

Rethinking Social Security

For a lot of good reasons—financial solvency, generational equity, realization of longer life expectancies, and encouragement of longer work lives—Social Security needs to be renovated. About $7 trillion of $22 trillion in future promises to beneficiaries are unfunded, not only for baby boomers but also for their younger brothers and sisters.[10] Even given that underfunding, returns on a beneficiary's lifetime contributions to the program are far less than people would voluntarily accept if it were, in fact, their own money. Further, the life expectancy, health status, and capacity of older Americans to work have all improved dramatically since the program was created in 1935.

When boomers begin looking closely at Social Security, they are going to discover a program designed for a completely different population and completely different economy than the one we have today. Social Security will be paying benefits to millions of boomers, such as Robert Smallwood, who will not need them, and paying inadequate benefits to those less-fortunate boomers, such as Avril Sanchez, who may have no other source of income, and funding all of those checks from the current incomes of young workers who are *certain* they will not receive benefits of comparable value when they reach eligibility.

The present Social Security system is biased toward pulling older workers from engagement in the workplace as early as age 62 toward a lengthy, socially subsidized holiday. And despite overwhelming indications that boomers plan on working past age 65, Social Security still discriminates against older workers. Though the Senior Citizens Freedom to Work Act of 2000 eliminated the older workers' earnings test after age 65 as a condition of receiving the benefit, it left in place punitive tax rates that reduce the benefit by one dollar for every two received for earnings over $10,000, in addition to the income and Social Security tax owed on the additional earnings.

Why the Scorched Earth Solution Won't Work

The catastropharian solution to the widening fiscal gap in Social Security is political poison and finds, predictably, few adherents in either the Republican or the Democratic camp—rapidly raise the retirement age to 70 or beyond, lift the ceiling on the least progressive federal tax (currently a flat 12.4 percent tax on the first $90,000 in wages annually, split equally between employer and employee), and means-test the benefits of higher-income beneficiaries, so that their benefits effectively disappear.[11] Toting up the political costs of this scorched earth solution, preternaturally cautious politicians could well conclude that the best course of action for them is to do nothing until something catches fire or until after *they* have retired, whichever is later. But there are other reasons besides political infeasibility why these are bad ideas.

Contrary to many experts, I believe that raising the age of eligibility for Social Security (and, more important, Medicare) is an inappropriate solution. Raising taxes on the wealthy is a venerable "class warfare" warhorse that both denies broad public ownership of the problem and glosses over the indefensible redistributive logic of the program. It isn't *merely* a funding problem to be corrected by "soaking the rich."

Means testing the benefit after a lifetime of "premium contributions" puts the lie to the social compact under which workers have supported the Social Security and Medicare systems.

Baby boomers have worked and contributed to the programs for a lifetime under the assumption—indeed, the legal guarantee—that they will eventually receive benefits based on their contributions to the program. Confiscating those contributions simply because an individual has worked hard and done well is an outrage. All workers have political "equity" in these programs and have a right to collect benefits they have contributed toward their entire lives.

The fact that Social Security is not now "on fire" presents an irresistible temptation to let the problems fester. If you believe that there is no problem with the current program other than that it does not take in enough revenues, the Democratic idea about abolishing the cap on the base salary against which the tax is levied makes perfect sense. If you are more ambitious and less partisanly political, however, a multiplicity of solutions is available.

New money will be needed to finance the two Social Security cash flow challenges: the 2017 crossover into red ink and, if you think, as I do, that they are a potential answer, the creation of private accounts. We can find five possible sources of these funds:

1. Unanticipated federal tax revenues from taxes paid by larger numbers of people continuing to work beyond age 65 (the baby boom's expected retirement delay)
2. Reduced cash outflows by voluntary deferral of Social Security payments by "well-reserved" or high-earning older baby boomers
3. Reduced cash outflows through reduction in the social "subsidy" paid to high-asset baby boomers when they finally enroll in Social Security
4. Money saved from phasing out the early eligibility option at age 62
5. A modest increase in the FICA deduction, devoted to funding private accounts

A major reason these solutions are not being discussed more broadly is that they do not fit the barren "tax the rich versus market solutions" dialectic of our current, political dialogue on the problem.

What Neither Party Wants to Do

Part I: Raise the FICA Deduction

The original purpose of Social Security was to increase the national savings rate to provide a secure foundation for older Americans. In the present inauthentic political discourse, whether Social Security continues to play a meaningful role in fostering national savings has somehow gone undiscussed.   If present national savings rates (presently zero) are inadequate, then returning to a discussion of the original purpose of the program might be timely.

Implicit in the Bush proposals was the idea that it was merely the rate of return on Social Security funds that was at fault. Those who believe in private accounts believe that individual investors should make the decisions that result in that increased return themselves and keep (and own) the resulting funds. Democrats argue that the Social Security tax system simply doesn't collect (and redistribute) enough. In the present political dialogue, the argument revolves around the extent and nature of the federal government's role, rather than whether we are saving enough.

Neither party wants to admit that, if the national savings rate is inadequate, then we need to modestly increase the tax rate and assure, rather than merely encourage, more savings. People who have been letting the appreciation in their home equity do their saving for them might well conclude, with the recent sharp downturn in home values, that they need to take a different approach. An obvious solution to the private-accounts funding problem is to distribute the pain of an increased savings rate across a large base of workers by both creating private accounts and funding them in major part through an increase in the payroll tax. If you believe the present savings rate of younger people is inadequate to build up a retirement cushion for them, and that Social Security is not, in fact, welfare but a social savings plan, then a more aggressive approach to mandatory savings might well be justifiable.

If it is clearly explained to voters that a modest increase in the payroll tax is required by our currently scandalously low national savings rate and *that they will own the additional dollars taken from their paychecks,* younger voters might tolerate the increase. The fact that significant numbers of young voters do not understand that they do not own their present Social Security benefits but would own the new accounts they are funding might also help build support for an obvious, if politically fraught, compromise between two currently irreconcilable positions.

Free market conservatives believe that increasing the payroll tax is coercive social policy and anti–job creation, because it invades the cash flow employers (who would have to match the increase) would have otherwise used to create new jobs. But if foreign or domestic investors do not wish to buy our equities or debt instruments because our society is looking more and more like a larger and glossier Argentina, at some not-so-magical point in the future, there will be no new jobs to argue about.

While we risk a confusing proliferation of tax-advantaged retirement accounts by creating new private accounts under Social Security, it may be worth the confusion if we can raise the current dismal savings rate.[12] The investment risk of these funds could be managed, per Kotlikoff, by insisting that they be invested in a handful of broad index funds, rather than individual stocks or mutual funds. The larger the cushion of private savings we can create for the "Might Be OK" forty-ish baby boomers, such as Peter Porter, the smaller the ultimate price will be paid in future public obligations subsidized by sharply higher taxes on younger workers.

Part II: Clarify Intergenerational Subsidies

The issue of sorting out who subsidizes whom is the festering core of Social Security reform. Some redistribution of incomes is inevitable in any social insurance scheme. Social insurance inherently redistributes incomes from young to old and from working to nonworking populations. However, how those subsidies operate is crucial, because it strikes to the heart of the social compact that Social Security represents. If the program is to remain universal, which I strongly advocate, then wealthy as well as poor people above a certain age should continue to be eligible for benefits. Everyone should have his or her lifetime contribution (their equity in the program) returned to them, with interest.

What wealthier retirees should not be entitled to is a subsidy from younger workers in excess of their contribution and a defined modest rate of return on their contribution (at least equal to the interest earned on the Trust Fund's notes). Many young workers paying into

Social Security and Medicare *know* they will never collect the level of benefits of today's retirees. Many of these younger workers also lack health insurance and private pensions. Today's young workers in benefit-free jobs are subsidizing the leisure and health care costs of retired doctors and investment bankers through their FICA and Medicare payroll deductions. They are, in fact, helping send Warren Buffett a Social Security check and paying a portion of his medical bills. Taxing these benefits as income diminished this problem somewhat, but did not banish it.

Transparency in intergenerational accounting is important for preserving public trust in the program. While some subsidy is an inevitable consequence of social insurance, it does not follow that all citizens are equally entitled to subsidy regardless of their income. Social Security is not "welfare"; it is a return of social capital that the federal government has borrowed, through a payroll tax, from the current population of workers.

Every American wage earner already receives a statement on his or her lifetime contribution to Social Security every year, as well as what he or she will receive when eligible for benefits. It is worth studying your statement the next time you receive one in the mail. The next, simple step in the process of making the system transparent is to show what percentage of the monthly benefit you will eventually receive is attributable to the your own contributions, what the investment return on your Social Security contributions has been over your working lifetime, and what percentage of your eventual check will have to come from others.

The final step in this process is to develop some logic that relates the level of social subsidy from younger workers in the beneficiary's check to the beneficiary's level of financial need. Conceptually, this preserves universality, because everyone, including the wealthy, will receive some level of Social Security benefit. The safety net character of the program will be as important to millions of "Struggling and Anxious" baby boomers, such as Avril Sanchez and should be strengthened through some form of a minimum Social Security benefit.

For these less-fortunate baby boomers, the subsidy from younger workers, as well as from working boomers should even be modestly increased to assure that they do not have to live in poverty. For those with substantial assets and private retirement funding, such as Robert Smallwood, however, the need for and claim on an intergenerational subsidy is hard to defend. The social subsidy part of their Social Security payment should be phased out for those whose incomes are above a certain threshold. For high-income retirees in 2010, this could represent as much as a third of their currently scheduled payment. Defining the appropriate rate of return on their lifetime contribution, as well as the income cut points for phasing out any social subsidy on top of their own contribution, will add administrative complexity to the program.

The bottom line is: the more fortunate boomers should receive smaller Social Security checks than they are entitled to under present law. The savings from this reduction in subsidy to the most fortunate boomers will go some distance toward closing the multitrillion dollar gap between future tax collections and promised benefits and also provide funding to assure that the least-fortunate baby boomers do not live the rest of their lives in poverty.

Withdrawing subsidies from higher-income older Americans is not a painless process; efforts to reduce subsidies of higher-income Medicare beneficiaries (by asking them to pay more of their health care costs) doomed the Medicare Catastrophic Coverage Act of 1988. However, I have yet to meet a single high-income boomer who has defended his or her right to a subsidized Social Security check when it is explained where the funds are coming from (e.g., their children). (Perhaps I have what statisticians call a "sampling problem.") The present method of taxing the benefit of higher-income Social Security recipients is a less-satisfactory method of achieving the same result, because the money reclaimed by income tax disappears into the maw of the U.S. Treasury. It would be a cleaner solution to exempt Social Security payments from taxation and restructure the benefit itself.

Some Social Security reformers have proposed an alternative strategy that produces somewhat the same result through a different means: switching the annual escalator on Social Security benefits from wages to prices (which rise more slowly than wages) and sheltering less-fortunate retirees from the diminished increase in their monthly checks.[13] This would result in less-fortunate retirees' receiving comparable checks to those provided them by the current law, while higher-income retirees receive somewhat less. However, this may not have the desired effect if tightening labor markets force wages up faster than prices in the coming labor market crunch discussed earlier.

The current level of checks to "Struggling and Anxious" baby boomers may not be adequate to keep them out of poverty. Increasing the amount of the eventual Social Security check received by low-income adults through a minimum benefit pegged to the poverty level and indexed to wage levels could assure that "Struggling and Anxious" baby boomers, such as Avril Sanchez, do not end up slipping into poverty as they age. Almost 10 percent of older beneficiary women, and 17 percent of unmarried older women, have incomes below the poverty level, as well as 24 percent of older African Americans and 19 percent of older Hispanics.[14]

Part III: Solve the "Retirement Age" Conundrum

Private accounts do not solve the problem of the advancing baby boom. To address this problem will require deciding whether we want to continue encouraging people to leave the labor market as early as age 62, as well as examining the timing of their eventual Social Security payments. The issue of tinkering with the age of eligibility for Social Security is complex and multifaceted. It is inappropriate simply to ignore the reality of the dramatic increase in life expectancy and, more important, the more dramatic improvement in the health status and work potential of people in their 60s and 70s. To leave in place a normative expectation that today's workers will spend a third of their lives in socially subsidized retirement is not defensible social policy.

As mentioned earlier, as a result of reforms enacted in 1983, the age of eligibility for Social Security is scheduled to rise to age 67 (in two-months-a-year increments) by 2027. For boomers born between 1943 and 1954, the age of eligibility for full Social Security benefits will be 66, not 65. Many policy makers conveniently out of the political firing line think this number should be 70 or 72 years old, and a good deal sooner than 2027. You won't hear a lot of talk about raising the retirement age during congressional or presidential election years.

The problem with raising the age of eligibility is simply that it will strand millions of "Struggling and Anxious" baby boomers who are likely to be unable to continue working to that age in a frightening limbo between work and Social Security (and, potentially, between private health insurance and Medicare). A politically formidable 15 million baby boomers, approximately 20 percent of the generation, have no private retirement funding and have an average net worth of $1,550 (excluding real estate assets), and will thus completely depend on Social Security.[15]

Many of these people are single women. Many less fortunate baby boomers will lose their jobs and be unable to find new ones before they reach age 65, let alone later. Many of the vulnerable "soon to be elderly" struggle, like Avril Sanchez, with disabilities such as alcoholism, depression, or debilitating lower back pain, or with the chronic disease challenges of diabetes and heart disease. Yet others are trapped by the moral imperative of caring for aging relatives and/or children and cannot work full time even if they are physically able.

Raising the age of eligibility for benefits without recognizing these limitations not only would be inhumane but also would result in a sharp and politically unacceptable rise in the poverty rate among older Americans. The group of baby boomers I am discussing is also likely to have higher than normal medical bills, particularly for prescription drugs. Raising the age of eligibility for Medicare, which is presently scheduled to remain at age 65, would create millions of new medically uninsured people.

There are already, inexcusably, almost 47 million people without health insurance in the United States, roughly 16 percent of the population. The practical result of raising the age of eligibility for Medicare for baby boomers would be to dump millions of poor and marginally unemployable people in their mid- to late 60s onto Medicaid rolls at a time when states will be struggling to control the growth of the program's expenses.

To address those who are unable to work and lack assets, some have suggested accompanying the increase in the age of eligibility for Social Security with a liberalization of eligibility for disability payments under Social Security.[16] There is some logic here. Disability payments, as defined by current Social Security law, are not age limited. Many current workers do not realize that they are eligible for Social Security disability payments decades before they are eligible for retirement benefits. Even more often, people apply for the benefit but give up early because they fail to understand the system.

From a fiscal standpoint, however, loosening eligibility standards for disability payments for the future surge of aging baby boomers would be like spraying kerosene on a raging fire. Disability outlays under Social Security are already skyrocketing, fueled by sharp increases in the numbers claiming disability. Total disability insurance program outlays increased from about $50.4 billion in fiscal year 1999 to about $70 billion in fiscal year 2003, while the number of workers and their dependents receiving disability benefits doubled from 3.9 million in 1985 to 8 million in 2004.[17]

Research has shown that more expansive coverage of disabilities coupled with weak earning opportunities for low-skilled workers has fueled this increase. Some policy analysts have speculated that laid-off or displaced workers used Social Security disability payments as a substitute for or supplement to unemployment insurance during the recent recession.[18] Disability payments may, in fact, be supporting a significant fraction of the nation's so-called discouraged workers, whose numbers do not figure in the unemployment statistics because many are not actively looking for work.

Altering eligibility standards for disability payments under Social Security simultaneous with the arrival of the baby boomers is like setting fire to your back porch to save the house; it merely relocates the fiscal crisis. It also invites the kind of legally sanctioned abuse currently seen among middle-class people who shed their assets to cover nursing home bills under the Medicaid program.

Phasing Out Early Enrollment and Deferring Benefits

An attractive alternative solution to the baby boom problem is to leave the present eligibility age (66 for early boomers and 67 for later boomers) where it is, but tinker with the incentives to enroll in the program. Currently, people can declare eligibility for Social Security as early as age 62, in exchange for a 20 percent reduction in scheduled benefits. This reduction is 13.5 percent if people retire at 63 and 6.66 percent if people retire at 64. A surprising proportion of people accept the early retirement option. Today, almost 70 percent of workers claim their Social Security benefit early, a number that has risen steadily over the past twenty years.[19]

The early enrollment option should be phased out over the next ten years, to reduce incentives for leaving the work force early. Those between 62 and 66/67 who cannot work should be encouraged to apply for disability coverage to smooth this transition. Those who continue working during this period but in low-wage jobs could be helped by making them eligible for the federal earned income tax credit. Eliminating incentives for early eligibility or sharply reducing the benefit workers receive when they do claim eligibility early is perhaps more important than raising the age of eligibility for full benefits, because it sends a signal that early eligibility is less appropriate now than it was when the option was created (in 1956 for women and 1961 for men).

For the tens of millions of baby boomers who continue working and are not likely to need their Social Security checks, strengthening the incentives to *defer* enrolling in the program is an excellent alternative to further increases in the age of eligibility for Social Security. There is currently an option, enacted in 1983, for potential beneficiaries to defer enrolling in Social Security to as late as age 71, in exchange for modestly increased monthly benefit payments (called "delayed retirement credits") when they do enroll. This option should be broadened and deepened.

Given that the *average* older boomer household will have more than $850,000 in household net worth by age 67 and that tens of millions of boomers will have private pension funding as well as "passive income" from investments, enhancing and lengthening the deferral option may make good sense for tens of millions of baby boomers. How much sense does it make to give them the benefit, and then tax away a big chunk of it because they have other income (earned or unearned), as is currently done? This large group of more-fortunate boomers ought to have choice and flexibility about when and how their Social Security benefit is deployed.

Lynn Etheredge, a policy analyst and former federal budget official, and Peter Orszag, an economist who is now chief of the Congressional Budget Office, proposed variations on a possible solution: replacing the delayed retirement credits with lump-sum payments of Social Security benefits. Upon reaching age 65, a baby boomer who wanted to continue working or who already had significant retirement savings and private health coverage could simply defer and receive the present value of benefits foregone in a single check, tax-free at the end of a year or multiple-year period of deferral. If a person deferred for a decade, for example, he or she would receive a lump sum at the end of the deferral period. This process is called "reverse annuitization."[20]

There could be a lot of options about how to deploy the lump-sum Social Security payment. The deferred payment would create financial options that a monthly check does not. Workers with 401(k) plans could roll this lump-sum disbursement into their 401(k) plan when they receive it. For people without private pensions, a lump-sum payment in lieu of monthly Social Security checks would create a new retirement asset that they could invest when they receive it. This option would work best for those who had low fixed expenses and who continued working at least part time. Etheredge showed that with a year's deferral of Social Security and Medicare, the federal government could write the "deferrer" a $10,000 check and make a "profit."[21]

There are attractive alternatives to the lump-sum payout option. One such alternative could be to extend the present deferred monthly payout option indefinitely, instead of ending it at age 71, with a higher level of ultimate benefit once the person enrolls in Social Security. Another and more cautious variation of the deferral approach, which saves significant money on current Social Security outlays, would be what Eugene Steuerle of the Urban Institute refers to as "back loading" the benefit—scaling Social Security benefit payments so that they start lower than they do now and increase as the worker ages. The logic here is that the longer the person lives, the higher his or her likely outlays for medical care and the greater his or her cash needs.[22]

It is possible that many baby boomers will guess wrong about their resource needs, outlive their pension and privately held assets, and face higher cash needs (e.g., for medical care) at the end of their lives than they do at 65 or 70. Back loading is another way of spreading out the Social Security obligation for the baby boom generation to accommodate this possibility. But it does not provide either the choice or the flexibility of the deferral approaches discussed earlier. Any of the deferral options generates current cash flow savings for Social Security by avoiding current payouts and gives the tax base and private market assets a chance to "grow into" the ultimate need.

It is conceivable that many millions of baby boomers, particularly those with significant savings or private pension resources, would elect to defer receiving their Social Security benefit, not merely until age 71, but into their early 80s. This end of the deferral period could be timed to the cessation of part-time work, or to the exhaustion of pension benefits, or to the onset of serious medical bills, or the requirement of long-term care.

As with all deferral options, the beneficiary is gambling that he or she will live long enough to receive the higher benefit. If the beneficiary dies before collecting the higher "ultimate" payment, as they say in poker, "the house wins," meaning that the government avoids having to pay any benefits for that person. (Gen X'ers and others who have not studied this issue closely perhaps do not realize that Social Security payments to the beneficiary cease on his or her death.) But because more than half of baby boomers who reach age 65 are likely to reach age 85, deferral at least into the mid-70s may not be a bad bet.[23]

A third possibility would be to give beneficiaries the option at age 66 or 67 to dedicate Social Security payouts free of tax to pay private long-term care insurance premiums. Present law enables beneficiaries to deduct Part B Medicare premiums from their Social Security checks, so the information technology is already in place to gather in the money. Currently, nearly half of the long-term care bill in the United States is paid for by individuals and families out of pocket. Medicaid pays most of the rest of the long-term care bill, in addition to providing medical services to the categorically needy. Medicaid has thus functioned for two generations as a publicly funded supplemental insurance program for long-term care.

To receive Medicaid benefits, middle-class families retain legal counsel and engage in creative divestiture of their assets until the target older person is "poor." This jury-rigged and demeaning process is not sustainable social policy today, let alone in twenty years. Medicaid benefits paid to middle-class homeowners who shift their assets to their children are not available to the truly needy, who remain among us and who were the intended primary targets of the Medicaid program in the first place. (The rules governing this "spending down" process were tightened significantly by the Deficit Reduction Act of 2005.)

While private long-term care insurance is broadly available, only about 10 million Americans have it.[24] The rate of growth has increased, particularly since the mid-1980s, but the proportion of the population age 50 or older with a long-term care insurance policy is still relatively small. In 2002 the U.S. Internal Revenue code was amended to provide for tax deductibility of employer contributions to long-term care insurance. There is no reason why baby boomers who have private pension coverage and savings could not be encouraged to deploy some of their Social Security benefit tax-free to pay private long-term care insurance premiums.[25]

The benefits in reducing future public outlays (e.g., Medicaid long-term care spending) could be considerable and might justify the loss in current tax revenue from not taxing the Social Security check. Another way to achieve growth in long-term care insurance coverage, which Etheredge suggested, would be to permit a portion of private pension funds to be "rolled over" into long-term care insurance premiums tax-free.[26]

Finally, for those "Set for Life" boomers, such as Robert Small-wood, who genuinely do not need the Social Security check, yet another option could be created for annual dedication of the "equity" amount of their Social Security payment to adopting an inner city school, or a national park, and to have the money transferred to an appropriate public purpose with a modest tax deduction to be applied against their other income.

Give Baby Boomers Choice and Control over Their Public Benefits

Baby boomers like choice and have insisted, particularly in regard to their health benefits and 401(k)s, on exercising control over decisions that affect their lives. This choice should be extended to how they receive the Social Security and Medicare benefits to which they are entitled as citizens and for which they have paid. Policy makers should leverage this revealed preference of baby boomers for choice into encouraging them to make choices about those public benefits that reduce or postpone federal spending where possible.

It is sensible public policy to "fuzzify" the use of age 65 as a boundary between work and retirement and encourage a lengthier work life. We need not only to create incentives for people to continue working but also to better integrate their publicly guaranteed benefits into their private savings and pension programs.

A flexible-benefits approach to Medicare and Social Security is permission-based and tailored to the specific needs of older Americans, working or not. Giving public benefits to people who do not need them in order to preserve an antiquated concept of uniform benefits is a waste of scarce public funds. Some of the resources created by deferral and reducing subsidies to the most fortunate baby boomers can be used to strengthen economic protection for the least fortunate members of the same generation, without adding to the fiscal overhang over subsequent generations. Taking advantage of the opportunity to reduce current outlays by providing benefits later in life and giving people options about how to deploy their benefits, properly done, is a win for everyone.

Social Security and Medicare are a vital part of the fabric of American society. That fabric should not be rigid and inflexible. Baby boomers come in all different shapes and sizes, and their needs differ dramatically. The United States remains a prosperous country. Resources are available to stretch these vital, publicly guaranteed benefits to better fit the diverse needs of a diverse generation. All that seems to be missing is the creativity and political courage to consider alternative approaches.

eight

What We Need to Do

At the beginning of this book, there were three stories of different baby boomers and their trajectory into the last third of their lives. The purpose of these fictional portraits was to illustrate the point that the baby boom generation is not monolithic and that the diversity of their circumstances will challenge policy makers. "One size fits all" solutions will not fit anyone well—hence, this book's emphasis on flexibility and personal choice within a universal social framework.

In this chapter, I consider how my recommendations might impact our three different groups of baby boomers. It has been argued that there are three broad groups of boomers, each comprising about a third of the generation. I called them "Set for Life," "Might Be OK," and the "Struggling and Anxious." Because these three groups require very different approaches, any social policy must be flexible enough to meet the needs of each group.

"Set for Life": Generating Capital for Tomorrow

The "Set for Life" group, represented by Robert Smallwood, was defined as baby boomers with deployable wealth, good health, and intellectual capital. These boomers are the driving force in the U.S. economy and society, controlling literally trillions of dollars in wealth as well as most of our corporations, universities, and nonprofit enterprises. Despite the glossy advertising images of healthy older Americans in *AARP, the Magazine,* they are not the majority of their generation, but they own the vast majority of its assets. They will play a strategic role in averting a fiscal "nuclear winter" for American society.

From a strategic standpoint, we want the "Set for Life" as well as their "Might Be OK" colleagues to continue working as long as they are vital and energized, well beyond age 65. Many will have the physical and intellectual potential to work well into their late 70s and early 80s, as such pioneering pre-boomers as Alan Greenspan, Warren Buffett, Bob Lutz, and Lena Horne have shown us. The revealed preferences for this group to continue working and investing will be the economic engine for continued growth in the economy and robust fiscal capacity for government.

As they work longer, they will supply positive social cash flow (taxes, capital investment resulting in job creation, etc.) from inside the baby boom generation itself to offset the costs we will inevitably incur taking care of their less-healthy and less-fortunate age peers. The reductions in social subsidy to high-resource baby boomers and the cash saved by their deferral of Social Security and Medicare benefits will help reduce their claim on scarce government dollars, while the earnings from their work and the enterprises they create will generate new tax revenues to help fund the needs of the less-fortunate members of their generation, in turn reducing the fiscal overhang onto Generations X and Y.

If the "Set for Life" do what they say they intend to do, there will be far more people over 65 with significant incomes than in the present. I differ from the catastropharians in believing that a far larger percentage of social needs of the baby boom generation will and ought to be self-financed, rather than shifted to younger people.

The "Set for Life" boomers will not actually need much help from government or society; they will use the degrees of freedom created by their wealth and knowledge to get what they want. What we need to do more than anything else is get out of their way—to eliminate barriers to their continuing to work, which they intend to do in any case, and to encourage them to continue creating new enterprises, both for profit and nonprofit, which can employ not only their own less-fortunate age peers but also younger people.

How can we encourage this trend? One way is to keep capital gains tax rates low to encourage enterprise formation and continued capital investment. We want the "Set for Life" boomers to deploy, not to sequester, their trillions of dollars in investment capital. We must also encourage employers to lengthen work careers, both by eliminating the remaining salary and pension policies that encourage retirement at or before age 65 and by creating flexibility for older workers to redirect their energies into new careers or flexible retirement.

In a "flattened" economy, to use Tom Friedman's phrase, upward mobility must be replaced by lateral mobility.[1] "Set for Life" baby boomers such as Robert Smallwood, who are already at the top of their respective fields, will benefit from policies that encourage "rewiring." They may not be influenced by the size of their pension payment, because they have extensive nonpension resources, such as real estate free of mortgage and private investment portfolios. What they are going to need most is continued intellectual challenge and opportunities to acquire additional skills and knowledge.

Complex and messy issues are raised by "Set for Life" baby boomers' access to public benefits. While they are unlikely to need their Social Security benefits, nearly all are going to need and use the Medicare program. At some not-so-magical point, no private employer or health plan is going to want to insure even the healthiest 77-year-old "Set for Life" baby boomer. Sooner or later, we're all going to be on Medicare. However, as has been earlier discussed, options for deferring the receipt of public benefits should be broadened and sweetened.

At age 66 or 67, or whatever age of eligibility Congress eventually legislates, more-fortunate baby boomers could simply elect to defer receiving Social Security and Medicare benefits. When they arrive at an age they choose, there would be a menu of options for deploying their Social Security benefits in a lump sum or else receiving higher monthly checks than those who did not defer. In the case of

Medicare, this incentive may take the form of reduced cost sharing or payment for services not otherwise covered by the traditional Medicare program.

What the "Set for Life" should not be entitled to is a social subsidy from younger workers or from the less-fortunate members of their own generation who continue working. Rather than receiving half again what they put into Social Security during their working lifetimes, high-income baby boomers should receive in benefits what they put in, plus an acceptable return on that capital. They should also pay a higher proportion of their own health care costs.

The "Set for Life" boomers will have substantial personal assets—current savings, investment portfolios, and private pension resources—that can sustain them. High-asset baby boomers should have the option of using their assets and resources, including Medicare payroll deductions received after age 66, to continue enrollment in private health care coverage that meets their needs. If they continue to work, payroll deductions taken from their paychecks after the age of eligibility for Medicare and Social Security could be used to subsidize private health care coverage or to purchase enhanced Medicare benefits, private long-term care insurance, or other, "gap filling" benefits as needed. To qualify for federal subsidy, these health plans should meet some minimal criteria for rewarding health care providers for maintaining continuing, health-promoting relationships with their "patients," most of whom are not actually "ill" at any one point and have robust disease-management program content.

Because Medicare is unlikely to evolve rapidly enough into a modern health-promoting health insurance plan that is transparent to the costs of care, keeping older workers in private health plans with health-promoting features, such as "consumer-directed" health plans, might accomplish more effectively the goal of keeping baby boomers healthier. Alternatively, many "Set for Life" boomers may find the simplicity of Part E Medicare benefit recommended earlier meets their needs better than continuing private health plan coverage.

"Set for Lifes" are also the health-obsessed segment of the baby boomer generation and the leading edge of "consumers" of healthy products and services, such as health spas and fitness centers. They have also catalyzed a boom in cosmetic surgical procedures, sports medicine, and other services that help people perpetuate the idea that they are really only 40. "Set for Lifes," particularly its women, have been the most aggressive and questioning health care consumers and have demanded that those who provide them care focus more of their attention on listening and meeting consumer needs. Whether this obsession with health and fitness will produce lasting results in improved function and quality of life will be interesting to study in future years. "Set for Lifes" will have the disposable income to pursue health promotion aggressively, as well as to pay more of their own health care bills.

Converting "Might Be OK" into "Set for Life"

The more "Set for Life" baby boomers there are, the better off the whole society will be. The only way to grow their numbers is to convert as many as we can of the "Might Be OK," the middle subgroup of baby boomers. The "Might Be OKs," such as Peter Porter, are that group of baby boomers who are currently "underreserved" for retirement, but who have the educational attainments and optimism to sustain longer careers and fill the resource gap. They currently lack sufficient private savings and free cash flow to enable them to retire when they wish to without suffering a sharp drop in their standard of living. They also face increasing burdens from obesity and obesity-related health risks, such as diabetes and heart disease. Because they have less disposable income, they are less likely than the "Set for Life" boomers to be aggressive consumers of spas, cosmetic surgery, and sports medicine but clearly feel societal pressure to live a more active, healthy life.

Even though most of them have secure jobs and current incomes, the "Might Be OK" members have fewer degrees of economic freedom than their "Set for Life" colleagues. They know they need to increase their savings, but a large number of the "Might Be OK" have difficulty supporting their current life-styles and financial obligations. They carry significant consumer debt and have harvested much of the growth in their home equity, the principal source of their wealth, by refinancing and spending the proceeds on current consumption or investments.

"Might Be OK" baby boomers lack the cash flow or resource cushion to take career or economic risks, or to take time off to acquire the new skills and knowledge that might enable them to move laterally in the economy. This is why employer investment in training and career development for older workers is particularly salient for the "Might Be OK" boomers. Policies such as paid sabbaticals and training opportunities for worker "rewiring" will help "Might Be OK" baby boomers to move laterally (or possibly upward) in the labor market. For self-employed "Might Be OKs," Achenbaum's idea of drawing on accumulated Social Security equity could make a strategic difference. The ability of boomers to take time off to reposition their careers without damaging current income or ultimate pension payouts will make a critical difference in creating more "Set for Lifes."

The most daunting barrier to self-employment is the cost, or even availability, of private health insurance for the self-employed. The inability of free agents to obtain health care coverage will introduce a lot of rigidity into the employment market for older workers and will inhibit lateral mobility that would otherwise occur. I earlier argued that the most efficient social means to do this is to disconnect the health benefit from employment and create a tax-based voucher system to fund health care coverage. Medicare coverage at age 55 could accomplish this disconnect for at least some older workers without raising taxes.

A major reason why "Might Be OK" boomers might not be OK is that their resources might not sustain the combined effect of income loss and out-of-pocket medical spending from a major illness. These risks increase as they enter Medicare, because of the substantial out-of-pocket exposure to health costs in the present program, as well as the chronic care expenses Medicare does not cover. Reducing this overhang by sensible redesign and simplification of the Medicare benefit, as with the Part E proposal, would resolve a major economic uncertainty for "Might Be OK" boomers. Extending the option of enrolling in Medicare down to age 55 might disproportionately benefit this group, if they could afford the premiums.

Measures to encourage increased saving will be vital to encouraging a buildup of resources for the "Might Be OK" baby boomers, so that they are less dependent on Social Security, or on their children, when they do wish to retire. Simply relying, as inertia and fantasizing would have it, on continuous appreciation in the value of residential real estate or equity portfolios is not sound social or personal planning.

While the reductions in taxes on dividends and capital gains enacted during the past six years may help increase private savings among "Might Be OK" boomers, eliminating these taxes for people below a certain income, say $200,000 a year, is a logical next step. The controversial policy of reducing or eliminating inheritance taxes, which will have the effect of passing through more of the trillions in inherited wealth baby boomer households have begun receiving from their parents, also has a role to play. While these may seem like expensive social gifts to the "Set for Life," continuing these tax reductions could make a difference to many marginally reserved "Might Be OKs."

There are legitimate objections that both tax changes shift the tax burden onto income and sales taxes, and therefore onto lower-income taxpayers who have no investment income, making the tax system even less progressive. Nevertheless, boosting private savings by a combination of personal financial discipline, compulsory savings in Social Security private accounts, and sheltering investment and inheritance income from tax is the only practical ways I can see of closing the retirement financing gap. With a little bit of luck, in the form of continued economic growth and a sustained rally in the stock market, increased savings on the part of "Might Be OK" boomers could translate into stronger family balance sheets and more "Set for Life" baby boomers.

The "Struggling and Anxious" Baby Boomers

The most serious challenge posed by the baby boomers for public policy, and for their families, resides in the "Struggling and Anxious" baby boomers, such as Avril Sanchez. The "Struggling and Anxious" boomers lack private savings and pension support and are spending every penny (and more) of their current earnings on current expenses, accumulating huge credit card and other consumer debt.

Unlike their "Might Be OK" colleagues, "Struggling and Anxious" baby boomers will find their health status or lack of skills limits their ability to work even to the current age of eligibility for Social Security and Medicare (on which they will be completely dependent), let alone to age 70 or 72. Indeed, many "Struggling and Anxious" boomers will find themselves "retired" by their employers due to poor productivity, caregiving obligations to struggling children, parents, or spouses, or limitations imposed by poor health, before they wish to retire. The size of this group will determine both the extent and the timing of the economic burden that the baby boomer generation ultimately imposes on society.

Reducing the size of this large and vulnerable group is one way to reduce the cost overhang onto younger workers and families, and it is the prime social policy imperative for anyone who worries about the future of this generation. To help the "Struggling and Anxious" will also require more effectively managing the health risks that could easily foreshorten their work careers and limit their life chances.

Chronic disease is our eventual lot in life and afflicts baby boomers in all different life situations. But many "Struggling and Anxious" baby boomers were already mired in chronic illness by the time they reach their early 40s. Many (though by no means all) of these diseases are among the most intractable and difficult in the spectrum of human illness, because they are rooted in addictions of various kinds (alcohol, tobacco, and other drugs). They are frequently compounded by depression, chronic pain from lower back problems, and arthritis. It is worth noting that many of these illnesses disproportionately affect those in lower socioeconomic strata, as well as minority groups. They are by no means the result exclusively of poor personal choices; in many cases, genetic inheritance or misfortune may be the cause. The least fortunate baby boomers are also those most likely to be obese, hence to be struggling with the onset of diabetes and respiratory and mobility problems.

While we can hope, in classic American fashion, for a pill that magically vanquishes these problems, the grim reality is that changing the behaviors at the root of these diseases is where the leverage is to improve the lives of the "Struggling and Anxious" boomers. It is difficult to imagine a more daunting challenge.

After nearly twenty years of being bombarded with messages from the media, friends, relatives, physicians, and others that smoking, drinking, eating fatty foods, and not getting enough exercise are bad for our health, a baby boomer would have to have been living in a cave or else been deeply inattentive not to have heard them. Unfortunately, our consumer culture has been sending baby boomers a different and much louder message for their entire conscious lifetimes. Large corporations have spent billions of advertising dollars "positioning" products such as cigarettes, beer, and cheap, carbohydrate-laden fast food as part of a modern life-style, beginning when consumers were children. As we now know, these products have barbed physiological hooks that hardwire their use into our neurochemistry and metabolism.

Some of the unhealthy habits reinforce one another. For example, people addicted to alcohol bulk up on the resultant carbs, contributing to extra weight or obesity. And when people cease smoking, as many adults who have shaken this habit have learned, they gain weight from enhanced appetite. Recent research estimated that as much as 20 percent of the recent weight gain in Americans was produced by the decline in cigarette use.[2]

Other health problems arise from failure to manage well-known health risks. Obesity contributes materially to the risk of diabetes, heart disease, and respiratory problems. People with these resultant illnesses can take statin drugs and beta blockers and can rigorously control blood sugar fluctuations with insulin. However, the root causes—poor diet and lack of exercise—stem from decisions people make every day that affect their health. Compromised access to preventive health care due to lack of health insurance has also played an important role in compounding those risks. As earlier discussed, while the poorest Americans have had access to medical care through Medicaid, the working poor and lower-middle class working in the unsheltered portion of the labor market (often in two or three jobs) frequently have not had health benefits.

Earlier Medicare coverage could play a crucial role in helping the "Struggling and Anxious" baby boomers get a handle on those health risks before they arrive at the conventional age of Medicare eligibility. As discussed earlier, this entrance would have to be publicly subsidized, as "Struggling and Anxious" boomers will not have the household cash flow to pay the premiums. Evidence suggests that better management of the known health risks of this 55–64 population could pay off in better health and reduced health costs when they do reach the traditional age 65 eligibility.

For those "Struggling and Anxious" boomers who do have health coverage through their employers, health-promoting corporate wellness programs have a major role to play in reducing the behavioral health risks that will lead to major social costs later. Yet the higher cost sharing associated with new "consumer-directed" health plans will put them out of reach for many cash-poor "Struggling and Anxious" boomers. These barriers could be reduced by restructuring cost-sharing and employer contributions in these plans to take into account the income of the worker and his or her family.

There is also a compelling case for encouraging more baby boomers, particularly the cash-poor "Struggling and Anxious" boomers, to join more traditional organized managed care systems such as Kaiser, whose current slogan is, most appropriately, "Thrive!" Because they appear to do a much better job of coordinating complex care and managing health risks, the much-misunderstood "managed care" plans—particularly the group and staff model variety—have major potential benefits for high-risk baby boomers. Improved access to primary care and the continuity provided by a "medical home" can most easily be provided in this type of health plan.

Even though baby boomers as a group detest medical paternalism, for some, a benign paternalism may be exactly what is needed. And for the "Struggling and Anxious" boomers, it is needed long before age 65. Hence, there is compelling public health logic to encourage boomers who take advantage of entrance into Medicare at age 55 to enroll in health-promoting private health care plans through Part C.

The goal of employers and health plans alike should be to encourage high-risk older employees to become "active agents" in improving their own health, not to discourage them from seeking preventive care early or from communicating with their primary care physicians. Increased cost sharing disproportionately affects the older, cash-poor "Struggling and Anxious" workers and families, who will have to divert funds from their grocery money to pay an increasing amount of their own care. This is why progressive employers have begun waiving cost-sharing for vital medications that reduce health risks as well as for some forms of preventive care.

Health-improving health plans are discovering that helping their subscribers connect the dots between their own behavior, compliance with the advice and medications their physicians recommend, and subsequent improvements in their health is an art form; many employees view the health plan not as a resource but as an adversary. It takes time, discretion, and thoughtful communication to help workers connect their own behaviors, particularly diet, exercise, smoking, and alcohol intake, as well as adherence to prescription drug regimens, to potential higher cash outlays and to provide them tools and help, through employee assistance programs, personal nurse programs, and other vehicles, to better manage their health risks.

Another potential leverage point for addressing the chronic illness of "Struggling and Anxious" baby boomers is the much-overlooked Veterans Administration (VA) health system. The VA is the largest organized health care system in the United States. Thanks to extraordinarily enlightened recent leadership during the past fifteen years, the VA has the most advanced information technology infrastructure of any major health care system in the nation, as well as one of the most rigorous clinical quality-assurance programs.[3] Almost no one outside the VA health system seems aware of these advances.

Vietnam veterans are overrepresented in the least-healthy fraction of the "Struggling and Anxious" population. Three million baby boomers and their older brothers and sisters experienced service in Vietnam, who are today in their 50s and early 60s. They returned not only with physical disabilities but also with addictions and catastrophic mental health problems that the VA was, at the time, woefully ill equipped to assist them with. By some estimates, 23 percent of the homeless population are veterans, and almost 50 percent of them served their country in Vietnam.[4]

The VA health system has struggled with how to stretch limited beds and medical professionals over a large population of eligible veterans, many of whom have asked the VA to cope with non-service-related disabilities and health problems. The VA has also had to cope with poorly defined boundaries with the privately and publicly insured health system.

The contemporary VA health system contains many of the tools to deal with the mounting toll of disability and chronic disease among the Vietnam veteran population, one of the highest-risk segments of the baby boomers. The VA probably has more expertise in coping with physical disabilities than the rest of the health system combined. It also lacks the "run the taxi meter" incentive of the private health system, because its physicians are salaried.

Developing the 24/7, "risk managing" clinical rationale I discussed earlier could pay big dividends in health improvement among this vulnerable Vietnam veteran population. Absent these efforts, we can anticipate a great deal of preventable illness streaming into hospital emergency rooms and a lot of Vietnam veterans who would otherwise be employable, tax-paying citizens becoming wards of the state.

The state is not the only social institution likely to be burdened by the rise in disability among the "Struggling and Anxious" baby boomers. Today more than 25 percent of Americans ages 18–34 live with their parents.[5] If they just stick around a few years longer, some Gen X'ers may make an unintentionally seamless transition from living with their parents as income consumers to living with their parents as caregivers. After a lengthy period of boomer parents' subsidizing their young, the "boomerang" Gen X'ers who returned home after college may find themselves caring for and supporting their aging and increasingly fragile parents.

Social subsidies will continue to play a large role in helping asset-poor baby boomers cope with eventual retirement. I earlier suggested that increasing the age of eligibility for Social Security strands a large number of "Struggling and Anxious" baby boomers. The risk of poverty among this population could materially be offset by establishing a higher minimum Social Security benefit, so that the least fortunate baby boomers are sheltered from economic hardship.

The "earned income tax credit" (EITC), which played a strategic role in facilitating the transition from welfare to work for younger people in the wake of the mid-1990s welfare reform,[6] could find new uses in helping "Struggling and Anxious" baby boomers. Through the income tax system, the EITC currently provides a worker with one child up to a $2,604 credit, which provides as much as a 34 percent matching subsidy, phasing out completely at a little more than $30,000.[7]

Subsidizing work for older Americans makes conceptual, labor market, and political sense. It could play a major role in weaning the older working population off of retirement subsidies as the principal income support.[8] Equally important, for those baby boomers who are being cared for by low-income children, extending the EITC to the children of ill or disabled parents could go a long way toward alleviating serious intergenerational financial burden.

Valid Social Policy Objectives

There is not going to be a "cure" for the mounting problem of age-related disability among baby boomers. In an important sense, aging is synonymous with rising disability. Cumulative disability, not acute illness, is the single largest problem the baby boomers will bring the health care system as they age. How we continue or accelerate the long-term trend of reduced disability among older Americans discussed earlier has particular saliency for the least fortunate third of the baby boom.

For the least-fortunate "Struggling and Anxious" baby boomers, the main barrier to continued engagement in work and community will be their health and the early onset of disabilities, many of which are not age-related. If we wait until the current age of Medicare eligibility to address these problems, we will have lost time and leverage to keep these boomers fit and employable.

The social payoff from postponing the onset of disability and managing its consequences is enormous—each individual boomer who can manage another five to fifteen years of at least part-time employment or volunteer activity will generate a large chunk of positive social capital (taxes paid plus public expense avoided), as well as minimizing the burden to his or her family. Living an active life and continuing to work, or to contribute as a volunteer, will help baby boomers both to remain connected and to minimize health care costs that their children would otherwise incur, as taxpayers and caregivers.

One Size Does Not Fit All

For baby boomers, a "one size fits all" social policy toward retirement will, emphatically, not fit all. Further, it will waste scarce societal dollars needed for younger people (education, human services) and for other pressing social needs (defense, homeland security, investment in science and technology, law enforcement, etc.). Further, a social policy designed for a different era and different economy will waste scarce dollars subsidizing people who are capable of contributing as well as taking care of themselves.

To create a pro-work, pro-health-improvement social policy will require social learning and a new concept of what it means to age. We do not want to subsidize a policy of segregating older Americans from the rest of society. It makes no sense for our modern society to finance a bright line between work and leisure that does not fit baby boomers' plans, self-concept, and values.

We should also not be subsidizing the leisure of baby boomers who have strong asset positions with scarce dollars squeezed from the paychecks of workers who do not have the margin to save for themselves. Being honest and transparent about who deserves social subsidies is an indispensable ingredient of a solution to this complex problem.

To the greatest extent possible, the strategies we choose must be permission-based, not coercive. They must rest on defensible incentives and signals to baby boomers to do things that are in the society's interest, as well as their own, particularly respecting their own health and financial well-being.

Perhaps in a time of political gridlock, ideological polarization, and short time horizons, it is asking too much of political leaders to create such a policy. But because most of them are baby boomers themselves and have family and personal stories replete with examples that illustrate the need for change, it may be easier than we think to create a social policy in which baby boomers and their younger fellow citizens both win.

nine

What Baby Boomers Should Do for Themselves

If we can say anything about baby boomers, it is that they have sought throughout their lives to control the things that affect them directly: career choice, personal relationships, health care, and health plan coverage. We should expect no different from them during the balance of their lives.

I have already discussed what public opinion data have told us about baby boomers' revealed preferences regarding their careers, retirement, income security, and the political system that guarantees them. I have analyzed the implications of these preferences for public and employer policy toward older Americans. In the previous chapter, I reviewed the effect of these policies on three large subgroups of boomers to help them reach their potential in the last third of their lives.

This chapter discusses what baby boomers should do to create choices for themselves in the next two decades. If you are a baby boomer, sensible personal choices made early can create significant degrees of freedom for the next twenty years and beyond. What are the most important choices, and how should you respond to them?

1. Start Something

Most baby boomers do not plan on ceasing working at age 65, though they may not continue what they have been doing for the past twenty years. Moreover, this may mean not salaried employment, but commitment to volunteer and community work. Almost 15 percent of boomers already plan on starting a new business or enterprise after age 65. More should do so.

Hence, the advice: Start Something. The Something may be a new business, or a new charitable enterprise, or a new division of an existing company, or a new product idea to be developed and sold to a potential commercial partner, or a new civic endeavor, or a new advocacy group, or a new neighborhood organization, or a new social or recreational club. These new enterprises will leverage personal relationships with age peers, family members, and younger colleagues at work. But new enterprises also create new relationships and extend social networks to those who share your passion.

Planning and creating new enterprises has the salutary effect of orienting the person forward and creates expectations of future performance that represent an alternative to self-indulgent consumerism or nostalgia. New enterprises consume energy (and often capital), but they also create new energy and, if they are successful, new capital as well.

Entrepreneurship is not just for the young. And entrepreneurship as a concept is by no means restricted to commercial activity. Social entrepreneurship creates social capital. Older experienced workers and citizens also bring a wealth of practical knowledge about people and their needs and about products and ideas that make them valuable as advisers, trustees and directors, angel investors, and counselors.

2. Become a Mentor to Younger People

Some of my mental health professional friends and colleagues believe that depression among older people, their principal so-called comorbid condition of any illness, may be the cumulative effect of grieving for lost friends and family members. As families have fragmented geographically, older Americans have also become more isolated. In a world of the extended family that lived in the same community, children and grandchildren were close at hand. As fewer boomers have formed families and have also moved away from the communities in which they grew up and from their own children, these sources of contact with younger people have withered away.

In an era of smaller and geographically diverse families, there is one obvious antidote to this inevitable thinning of our peer group: creating new relationships with younger people through work, professional, or philanthropic activities, volunteering or recreational activity, hobbies or other common interests. Being a mentor is a lost art; once institutionalized in such roles as apprenticeship, mentoring is an extraordinarily valuable method not only of transmitting knowledge but also of sharing power with younger people.

Mentoring has the important collateral benefits of diversifying the age mix of our colleagues and friends and of exposing the mentor to new ideas and learning from younger colleagues. Multiplying relationships and diversifying them across the generations is an important way to remain connected to our communities and to others and of avoiding the turning inward that all too often characterizes aging.

3. Pick a Single Focal Point for Health Care Interactions

Our medical care system has a reflexive tendency to subdivide us into organ systems and assign a specialist to guard each organ. In this default medical world, the whole person has no organic reality and ends up being a great deal less than the sum of his or her parts. If we have the time and patience to manage all the relationships, we can, as we age, end up with a dozen or more physicians, each of whom has a special relationship with a piece of us—one for our heart, another for our nervous system, a third for our bones and joints, a fourth for our kidneys, a fifth for our ears, nose, and throat.

Outside of well-organized medical group practices or group-model health plans, such as Kaiser, it is unusual for all these multiple physicians to communicate with one another or even to be aware that other physicians are involved with "their" patient; each physician busily addresses a focused area of expertise as if the other physicians and their care plans did not exist. This medical pluralism is the explanation for the several dozen medicine bottles one finds in a typical older person's medicine cabinet, a systemic hazard of aging independent of our actual health.

There are wonderful exceptions to this process. The Mayo Clinic, for example, designates a single physician as the point person for a diagnostic evaluation, orchestrating the activities of all consultants and framing the decisions patients need to make. Consultants in Mayo's system gracefully and willingly submit to "coordination" by this single physician and act in a supporting role. In most of its regions, Kaiser Foundation Health Plans assign a single, primary care provider the responsibility for continuity of relationships with older subscribers.

As a centerpiece of the needed redesign of Medicare, I recommended that Medicare encourage its beneficiaries to pick a "medical home"—a single physician or other health care provider as the focal point for all medical care. Relationship-based payment fosters the development of a focal point for an older person's medical care.

Even if Medicare is not redesigned, however, there are important reasons for individuals to adopt this approach to managing their own health care. Perhaps the most important reason for doing this is that if one does not, the responsibility for managing your care at some point will almost inevitably devolve onto a family member, who may have other ways they wish to spend their time.

Training that single informed decision maker for older people has been the objective for the perpetually emerging medical specialty of geriatrics. Geriatricians are specially trained in the medical as well as social needs of older people and integrate that knowledge across medical disciplines to advocate for improved health of their patients. Geriatrics has struggled to gain acceptance and legitimacy in a specialty-dominated health care world. It has special relevance for the quality-of-life concerns of baby boomers as they age.

If good medicine is, at base, a productive exchange of knowledge between the patient and the health care providers, finding a focal point for that knowledge seeking and transmitting is very important.

If we do not make explicit the responsibility of some health professional to see the whole playing field when we are older, we are going to receive suboptimal medical care and expose ourselves to needless risk from a poorly organized response to our needs.

4. Anticipate End-of-Life Decisions

This is one area in which baby boomers' penchant for wishful thinking works against them. Baby boomers will control many things in their lives, but almost certainly not the time or circumstances of their own death. Moreover, not all of us will go as perhaps some of us fantasize—quickly and painlessly.[1]

The Terri Schiavo case provided a well-timed and grisly example of what happens when a person is incapacitated by illness before she can declare what she wishes her family and the health care system to do in respect to end-of-life care. The political and legal circus of the Schiavo case should be a cautionary tale to boomers that we may not like the decisions that end up being forced on our families if we do not provide them explicit written guidance about what we want to happen to us.

We now know that the default setting of both the health care system and an influential wing of our political system is to continue to maintain a person indefinitely even if he or she is hopelessly impaired and not capable of returning to a satisfying or productive life. The most important incapacity may be not physical, but a loss of memory and cognitive function.

Because so many baby boomers are currently experiencing this dilemma with their own parents, they have no valid excuse for not having living wills that specify how they want end-of-life decisions to be handled and, equally importantly, durable powers of attorney, to enable a trustee or loved one to make financial decisions if they are incapacitated and cannot make decisions for themselves. These experiences with our parents provide us not only useful guidance for how we want the ends of our own lives to be different but also the motivation to make those desires explicit.[2]

Several steps are necessary before creating the legal documents: decide what you want to happen in the eventuality that you become irretrievably ill, have a dialogue about these choices with someone you trust, and secure this person's agreement to act on your behalf. One important component of this is to empower someone to seek palliative care, such as hospice care, as an alternative to curative medicine.[3] Public policy is still evolving in this area, as the recent Supreme Court consideration of assisted suicide illustrated.[4] If we do not overcome the baby boomer predilection for spontaneity on this issue, we will inexcusably create painful dilemmas and decisions for our families.

5. Purchase Long-Term Care Insurance

Another area in which the baby boomer predisposition to wishful thinking will hurt us is in failing to plan for long-term care. Medicare covers long-term care, particularly home care, skimpily at best. The basic principle of Medicare was to cover long-term care needed to recover from an episode of illness, a worthless concept in dealing with chronic disease. As a result, Medicare covers only a fraction of the care needs of an aging person.

Only about 10 million Americans currently have private long-term care insurance coverage. The rest of us are placing our estates and loved ones at risk by not having it. Though it is possible to begin coverage in our 60s (providing we are in reasonable health at the time of enrollment), the best value is to establish coverage while in our late 40s or early 50s.

In 2003 Congress amended the Internal Revenue Code to make long-term care insurance a deductible business expense, encouraging employers (including the self-employed) to purchase it. If your plans include leaving assets to your children, purchasing long-term care insurance is a way of protecting those assets from the virtually uncontrollable risk of lingering chronic care expenses.

6. Don't Settle for Obesity

Approximately 30 percent of the adult population of the United States is obese. While there are encouraging signs that adult obesity is leveling off, a large fraction of baby boomers are going to be markedly increasing their health risks by remaining obese. Along with the rising intake of empty calories from soft drinks and snack food, the lack of physical activity has been the principal culprit in the rising level of obesity in American society.

The tragedy is that the single most effective thing we can do to avoid obesity costs nothing and involves doing something pleasurable. It doesn't take five 90-minute aerobics classes a week to fight this problem; a 30-minute walk every day after dinner has a surprisingly salutary benefit.

According to the Centers for Disease Control (CDC), a regular, preferably daily regimen of at least 30 minutes of brisk walking, bicycling, or even a mundane activity, such as working around the house or yard, will reduce your risks of developing coronary heart disease, hypertension, colon cancer, and diabetes.[5] It may be the single highest-leverage way of postponing the onset of chronic illness. There are also social benefits from extending the dinner hour and coming into contact with neighbors and friends.

Controlling the intake of refined sugar and reducing the intake of carbohydrate-laden "empty calories" also has a major contribution to make in bringing obesity under control. Cynthia Kenyon, the University of California geneticist who unlocked the genetic secret of how to achieve a sixfold increase in the life-span of the *C. elegans* roundworm, made one important modification in her own diet as a result of her scientific discovery: she sharply reduced her intake of refined sugar (such as high-fructose corn syrup found in soft drinks, breakfast cereal, cookies, and snack food).[6]

7. Don't Be a Lazy Saver

Baby boomers are saving for retirement at approximately the same rate as their parents and have a better asset position than their parents did at this stage of their lives. But overall savings rates in our society, including baby boomer younger siblings and children, are far too low for the U.S. economy to be sustainable in the long term. We need to raise the savings rate, and doing this will require creating positive cash flow in our household budgets. If we cannot do this, our dollars may no longer be hard currency should we wish to spend them overseas.

Baby boomers have lived through a remarkable twenty-year period in which they could let their stock portfolios or the rising values of the homes they live in do the saving for them (though the rising home prices appear to have reversed by the end of this writing project!). Rising asset values may be a casualty of a smaller group of prime earners (as Gen X'ers will become). Boomers who continue relying on passive asset appreciation as their principal saving mechanism are exposing themselves to excessive economic risk, especially in the event of an economic downturn.

The only sure way to save is to spend less every month than you are taking in. As baby boomers near retirement, they are going to need to pay down mortgages, consumer loan balances, and car payments to the point where they can live on what they earn plus what they receive from pensions and Social Security. Reaching the point of positive cash flow earlier than retirement is the key to not having a sharp decline in standard of living when they do cease working.

I've read a lot of books on this daunting subject. By far the best has been Lee Eisenberg's *The Number: A Completely Different Way to Think about the Rest of Your Life*.[7] Eisenberg has thought a lot about the social and emotional reasons why people do not plan financially for the rest of their lives, and he addresses a complex topic with both dry wit and rigor.

Optimism Is Not a Strategy

Baby boomers bring to the last decades of their lives a lot of positives: optimism, a sense of efficacy, curiosity, an intense work ethic, technological prowess, high education levels, and a high level of interest in health issues and in controlling decisions that affect their health. These are vital ingredients of a successful last third of life; they are self-generators of energy.

As difficult as it may be for baby boomers to accept, we are not going to be able to control everything that happens to us in the latter phases of our lives. Merely hoping for the best, while ignoring the future consequences of decisions we postpone making today, is going to be an unsuccessful recipe for a happy aging process.

Eventually, aging is going to limit baby boomers' options and possibilities. And, at a time and place not of our choosing, we will all die, however young we may feel today. In contrast to our accepting parents and grandparents, baby boomers have been activists and have defined what they want to accomplish in every phase of their lives so far. Taking active steps that create options in the next twenty years will pay enormous dividends in life satisfaction and renewed and strengthened relationships.

Conclusion

Predicting the future is fraught with risk—the ever-present danger of being embarrassed by the unfolding of actual events. Nevertheless, people seem morbidly fascinated by forecasters and our frail arts. Compelling visions of the future have a self-fulfilling aspect. This is because expectations are a powerful engine of behavior change, perhaps the most powerful of all.

Almost a century ago, the so-called Chicago School of sociology proposed a central organizing principle of human behavior called the Thomas Theorem (after W. I. Thomas): when a situation is defined as real, it is real in its consequences. The same principle underlies a school of economics, from the selfsame University of Chicago, called "rational expectations," or RatEx, which argued that investors make investment decisions based on their expectations of future economic conditions. When someone shouts "fire" in a crowded theater, the fire may be illusory, but the stampede and crushed bodies are all very real. This is why we need to be careful not to shout "fire" upon the mere smell of smoke. Shouting "fire" is exactly what our catastropharian friends are doing regarding the fate of the baby boom generation.

I love rivers. There is a reassuring inevitability to what they do, and they make a mesmerizing sound. One of my favorite leisure-time pursuits is running rivers, both white water rafting and kayaking. An interesting discovery I have made about running rivers is that when one spots a large hazard downstream, such as a huge, gnarly rock or a seething whitewater hole, focusing obsessively on it is an almost surefire recipe for running right into it and taking a cold, bruising swim.

We are in serious danger of doing this as a society with the aging of the baby boom generation. In a singularly unimaginative and depressing fashion, catastropharians see baby boomers following the life trajectories of their less-educated and less-energetic parents and grandparents, retiring en masse at age 65, and moving to Florida or Nevada to play golf and evening canasta.

The purpose of this book has not been to demonize retirement. Many boomers will do exactly this. Eventually all of us will gear down, either voluntarily or involuntarily, because we will no longer desire or be able to work. Some baby boomers who work in boring or onerous jobs have been looking forward to and saving for retirement. We do not want to devalue boomers' personal choices by penalizing them economically or stigmatizing them socially when they do.

A large fraction of baby boomers, however, have other plans, and their expressed desires provide guidance on how we should begin rethinking our social policy toward older Americans. Those expressed desires are potentially highly beneficial to society as well as to them. We should begin resetting our social expectations to encourage a more active and healthier last third of life and actively support their aspirations by changing our public policies toward older people.

Along the way, there are problems that need solving. Many baby boomers lack adequate private savings and have less than optimal personal health habits. In both cases, these problems originate in a lamentable tendency to trade present pleasures against future security and health. Failure to address these concerns will impose future costs on the society and on the baby boom itself in avoidable health care bills and in income-security needs. Put more positively, the healthier and more solvent baby boomers are, the smaller the social burden they will impose in the next twenty years.

This book has urged that we create a pro-work, pro-savings, pro–health improvement social policy for baby boomers and those who come after them. We need to change the signals embodied in current employment and tax policies to encourage those who are able to and interested in working to continue doing so.

This book has focused on the outlook for baby boomers over the next twenty years. There is no question that *whenever* baby boomers do cease working, American society is going to incur significant costs, in both social support and medical expense, of managing the end-of-life costs of the baby boom generation. My purpose has been to remind readers that baby boomers, who are currently between ages 44 and 62, have degrees of freedom to address their own (and society's) problems in important ways that can avert or moderate, perhaps for a generation, a potential fiscal and social crisis.

Catastrophe is far from inevitable. Demography is not destiny. We have lots of room to make intelligent social and personal choices to create a happier and more prosperous society. Better health of older Americans, a changed work world, and the desire of baby boomers to continue working all point to a far better near-term outcome than most social observers believe. Encouraging longer and more productive engagement of older Americans in work as well as in their communities and postponing the onset of serious, life-changing illness are both big wins for American society.

As we reach the decade of the 2030s, the youngest baby boomers will turn 65 and the oldest will be in their middle to upper 80s. Unless there are remarkable advances in the treatment of degenerative diseases, a large and mounting burden of unavoidable health care costs will weigh down American society. While a third or more of the baby boom generation could still be working in the year 2030, a larger number will be dependent on their own asset base and on our social programs.

The shape of the health care system and society in 2030 and after is legitimately the topic of another book. But the shape of the 2030 disease burden is less mysterious, because epidemiological trends change much more slowly than biomedical science does; the front end of 2030's disease burden is already visible to us. It is going to be, by any measure, hugely expensive to address. Health care costs we have successfully postponed in the next twenty-five years begin coming due in this complex decade.

Growth: The Indispensable Ingredient

The debate over what to do about the longer-term problem the baby boom poses should not only encompass how to make health care more affordable and the appropriate roles of the home, family, and community in caring for baby boomers but also focus on the type of economy and society we need to finance that burden. A growing, vital country of 400 million people will have more degrees of freedom to cope with this burden than a stagnant, depressed country of 320 million. As a recent *Wall Street Journal* editorial put it, "Paying benefits to 75 million baby boomers in 2030 will be a much lighter lift if we have a $25 trillion GDP and a net worth of $100 trillion than if slower growth in the interim years leaves us, say, a third less wealthy."[1]

We will find some clues about this tension between the "costs" of an aging population to society and how important economic growth is in managing them from our European colleagues. In Europe, not only do its societies contain a higher proportion of older people than American society does, but its economies, with some exceptions (Britain, Spain, Ireland), are also not growing nearly fast enough to cushion the fiscal blow. Because the pressures are unavoidable, these countries will alter pension policy and their largely socialized health care systems before we do.

Counting on Continued Economic Luck

We certainly do not control all the factors that sustain future economic growth. Even those economists with stellar academic credentials and forecasting track records would be hard pressed to forecast a twenty-five-year economic future as rosy as our past twenty-five years' growth. If we have only one significant recession in the next twenty-five years, we will be astonishingly lucky. The most serious downside risk of globalization is that because the U.S. economy is so tightly wired to that of the rest of the world, significant economic problems anywhere in the world can have an instant and negative effect on our well-being.

It is also a dangerous world. The United States has resourceful enemies who wish us harm and who have struck us both at home and abroad. Successful radical Islamic risings in currently friendly countries or a general war in the explosive Middle East could destabilize our economy, as could an economic collapse or political instability in China. These and other uncontrollable risks impose costs in economic uncertainty, and thus affect the cost of energy, interest rates, food and medicine, and a host of other important economic factors. Resulting damage to our equity markets would move a lot of thinly capitalized and poorly hedged baby boomers right back into economic danger.

Finding the Virtuous Cycle and Riding It

While we cannot control these external risks, we can mitigate some of their effects by better planning and integration with our international partners. We will have fewer excuses, however, for failing to capitalize on the positive momentum inside our own borders. Americans should begin developing a culture and economy more supportive of older people who wish to continue to work or contribute actively to their communities in other ways. We can also do a much better job of anticipating and managing the health risks that affect older Americans.

If we use our collective imaginations, we can design alternatives to a stagnant, age-segregated society and interrupt the vicious cycle of disengagement, deteriorating health, and depression that can, all too often, accompany aging. This book has suggested that, if we are imaginative, we can design and reinforce an alternative, virtuous cycle: education and new knowledge create new work roles and a more active, engaged life, which in turn generates positive health effects that enable people to work and create longer and generate the curiosity and energy to seek more new knowledge. By reinforcing that virtuous cycle, we can postpone and spread out the social costs of the baby boom.

From a fiscal standpoint, new migrants to the United States and the echo boomers are like the cavalry riding to the rescue of our economy. Unlike our unfortunate colleagues in Europe, whose populations are declining and many of whose economies are stagnant, Americans have continued a remarkable run of economic growth. Though we owe much more than we should to foreign governments because we have not saved enough publicly or privately, we have degrees of economic freedom other societies do not have to solve our generational problems.

Whether our political system is flexible enough to permit these changes is an open question. The recent, interest group–dominated attempt to reform the Medicare program (in 2003) and the bitterly polarized nondebate over Social Security reform are not encouraging signs. They suggest an inability or unwillingness of our politicians to transcend a stale seventy-year-old "market versus social democracy" political dialectic. A thoughtful response to the challenge of an aging baby boom is not about markets, or about generational equity, or preserving the New Deal. It is about what we need to be a productive, growing, and sustainable economy and a humane, vital society.

In a democracy, as Winston Churchill reminded us eighty years ago, we get the government we deserve. In a free society, we get the future we deserve. By denying the need to make conscious social and personal choices, we postpone the difficult decisions—for example, reallocating subsidies, increasing social and personal saving, increasing transparency and accountability for health care costs, and improving our own health. Neither the glacial pace of demographic change nor the seemingly glacial accretion of physical limitations related to aging provides an immediate stimulus to action.

What we baby boomers need to do is ask ourselves an important question: given what we have witnessed of the end of our parents' and grandparents' lives, what would we do differently for ourselves? If we begin working now to create a different life path, we can create degrees of freedom unimagined by our elders, lives we can be proud of and an end of life that we can accept with grace.

Notes

Introduction

1. L. J. Kotlikoff and S. Burns, *The Coming Generational Storm: What You Need to Know about America's Economic Future* (Cambridge, Mass.: MIT Press, 2004), pp. xvii–xviii.

2. C. C. Mann, "The Coming Death Shortage," *Atlantic Monthly* 295, no. 4 (2005): 102.

3. G. Easterbrook, *The Progress Paradox: How Life Gets Better While People Feel Worse* (New York: Random House, 2003).

One • The Baby Boom

1. National Center for Education Statistics, U.S. Department of Education, *Education Statistics Quarterly* 1, no. 1 (Spring 1999).

2. Bureau of the Census, Census Questionnaire Content, 1990 CQC-13 (1990).

3. W. H. Frey, "Institute Review: Boomers in the 'Burbs," *Milken Institute Review,* no. 2 (2000): 85–91.

4. Bureau of the Census, Census Questionnaire Content, 1990 CQC-13.

5. Frey, "Institute Review: Boomers in the 'Burbs."

6. J. H. Makin, "Oil and Stagflation," American Enterprise Institute for Public Policy Research, *Economic Outlook,* AEI Online Publication, September 2004, p. 1.

7. E. Taylor, *Prime-Time Families: Television Culture in Postwar America* (Berkeley: University of California Press, 1989).

8. J. Leeds, "Iron Man Slows, and So Does the Industry," *New York Times,* June 25, 2006.

9. L. Steinhorn, *The Greater Generation: In Defense of the Baby Boom Legacy* (New York: St. Martin's Press, 2006).

10. Boston Women's Health Book Collective, *Our Bodies, Ourselves* (New York: Simon and Schuster, 1970).

11. Lt. Gen. Barry R. McCaffrey, Assistant to the Chairman of the Joint Chiefs of Staff, speech to Vietnam veterans and visitors gathered at "The Wall," Memorial Day 1993. Reproduced in the *Pentagram,* June 4, 1993.

12. See J. Todd, *Desertion: In the Time of Vietnam* (New York: Houghton Mifflin, 2001), for the story of one of these expatriates.

13. D. P. Moynihan, *Family and Nation: The Godkin Lectures, Harvard University* (New York: Harcourt Brace Jovanovich, 1986).

14. D. Coupland, *Generation X: Tales for an Accelerated Culture* (New York: St. Martin's Press, 1991).

15. C. Davies et al., "A Changing Political Landscape as One Generation Replaces Another" (Washington, D.C.: AARP, 2004), p. 6.

16. J. Love, "Political Behavior and Values across the Generations: A Summary of Selected Findings," AARP Strategic Issues Research (2004). http://assets.aarp.org/rgcenter/general/politics_values.pdf.

17. Ibid.

18. C. Davies and J. Love, "Tracing Baby Boomer Attitudes Then and Now: A Comparative Look at the Attitudes of Baby Boomers in the 1970s and 2002," AARP Knowledge Management, August 2002. http://assets.aarp.org/rgcenter/general/bbattitudes.pdf.

19. C. Keegan et al., "Boomers at Midlife 2003: The AARP Life Stage Study; Research Report" (Washington, D.C.: AARP, 2003).

20. U.S. Congress, Congressional Budget Office, "Baby Boomers' Retirement Prospects: An Overview," November 2003. www.cbo.gov/showdoc.cfm?index=4863&sequence=zero.

21. J. Gist and K. Wu, "The Inequality of Financial Wealth among Boomers," AARP Public Policy Institute Data Digest, July 2004. www.aarp.org/research/assistance/incomedist/aresearch-import-885-DD100.html.

22. C. Keegan et al., "Boomers at Midlife 2004: The AARP Life Stage Study; Research Report" (Washington, D.C.: AARP, 2004). www.aarp.org/research/reference/publicopinions/Articles/aresearch-import-931.html.

23. S. Zapolsky, "Baby Boomers Envision Retirement II: Survey of Baby Boomers' Expectations for Retirement" (Washington, D.C.: AARP, 2004). http://research.aarp.org/econ/boomers_envision.pdf.

24. Ibid.

Two • The Social Safety Net for Older Americans

1. U.S. Department of Agriculture, Economic Research Service, *Farm Policy, Farm Households, and the Rural Economy: Agricultural Policy Tools and Objectives,* July 2005. www.ers.usda.gov/Briefing/Adjustments/policytools.asp.

2. A. M. Schlesinger, *The Crisis of the Old Order, 1919–1933* (New York: Houghton Mifflin, 1958).

3. W. A. Achenbaum, *Social Security: Visions and Revisions*, A Twentieth Century Fund Study (Cambridge: Cambridge University Press, 1986), p. 16.

4. Ibid.

5. National Center for Health Statistics, *National Vital Statistics Reports* 52, no. 3 (September 18, 2003). www.cdc.gov/nchs.

6. Information Please Database, "Educational Attainment by Sex, 1910–2004," Pearson Education, Inc. (2005). www.infoplease.com/ipa/A0779809.html.

7. Achenbaum, *Social Security*, pp. 18–28.

8. Ibid., p. 23.

9. Social Security Online, "Frequently Asked Questions." www.ssa.gov/history/age65.html.

10. Achenbaum, *Social Security*, pp. 32–33.

11. Ibid., pp. 43–44.

12. A. M. Schlesinger, *The Coming of the New Deal, 1933–35* (New York: Houghton Mifflin, 1958), pp. 385–406.

13. J. A. Poisal, C. Truffer, S. Smith, et al., "Health Spending Projections through 2016: Modest Changes Obscure Part D's Impact," *Health Affairs* (Web Exclusive) 26, no. 2 (2007): W248.

14. Pew Research Center, "Who Votes, Who Doesn't and Why," October 18, 2006. http://people-press.org/reports/display.php3?ReportID=292.

15. E. Porter, "Coming Soon: The Vanishing Work Force," *New York Times*, August 29, 2004.

16. See J. Goldsmith, "47 Million Hostages," *Health Affairs* online, September 13, 2007, for discussion of the diversity of the uninsured population and the political difficulties it presents. www.healthaffairs.org/blog/09/13/.

17. T. R. Marmor and J. L. Mashaw, "Fact and Fiction: The Contemporary Attack on Social Insurance in the United States," paper presented at the 2nd International Research Conference on Social Security Organized by the International Social Security Association, hosted by the National Insurance Institute, Jerusalem, Israel, January 25–28, 1998.

18. J. Love, "Political Behavior and Values across the Generations: A Summary of Selected Findings" (Washington D.C.: AARP, 2004), p. 9.

19. Democracy Corps, "Getting the Public to Listen," February 28, 2007. Special analysis of age patterns provided by Avi Zollman, September 10, 2007.

20. S. Zapolsky, "Baby Boomers Envision Retirement II: Survey of Baby Boomers' Expectations for Retirement" (Washington, D.C.: AARP, 2004).

21. D. Walker, Controller General of the United States, "Fiscal and Healthcare Challenges," presentation to Marwood Group, April 25, 2007.

22. A troublesome exception is payments for physician services under Part B, which were capped in 1997 to grow at a rate tied to GDP growth, through a formula based on a so-called sustainable growth rate (SGR). This formula reduces physician fees automatically when growth in Part B expenditures exceeds the

SGR. Congress has overridden these reductions almost every year since the formula went into effect.

23. The original age of eligibility for Social Security was gradually increased from age 65 by the Social Security Amendments of 1983. See Achenbaum, *Social Security*, pp. 81–99, for the legislative history of this change.

24. OECD Statistics, "OECD Statistical Profile of Germany, 2006." http://stats.oecd.org/WBOS/ViewHTML.aspx?QueryName=182&QueryType=View&Lang=en.

25. Poisal et al., "Health Spending Projections through 2016."

26. L. J. Kotlikoff and S. Burns, *The Coming Generational Storm: What You Need to Know about America's Economic Future* (Cambridge, Mass.: MIT Press, 2004), p. 51.

27. Ibid., pp. 42–44.

28. Older people are not the sole beneficiaries of either program. According to the 2004 Report of the Trustees of Social Security, 7 million survivors of deceased Social Security beneficiaries and 8 million disabled workers and their dependents received Social Security benefits in 2003. Many of these beneficiaries are younger than age 65. Further, long-term Social Security disability recipients under age 65, as well as dialysis patients, receive Medicare benefits. Nevertheless, supporting older people is the core business of both programs. See "The 2004 Report of the Board of Trustees of the Federal Old-Age and Survivors Insurance and Disability Insurance Trust Funds." www.ssa.gov/OACT/TR/TR04.

29. At least one catastropharian novel has dramatized the political moment when younger people wake up to this reality: Christopher Buckley's *Boomsday* (New York: Hachette Press, 2007). The book is highly recommended.

30. See Christine Cassel's *Medicare Matters: What Geriatric Medicine Can Teach American Healthcare* (Berkeley: University of California Press, 2005), for an eloquent statement of this argument.

31. "Social Security Poll Otherworldly," *Wisconsin State Journal*, March 19, 1997, p. 11A.

32. U.S. Census Bureau, Income, "Poverty and Health Insurance Coverage in the US, 2006." www.census.gov/prod/2007pubs/p.60-233.pdf.

33. U.S. Census Bureau, "Census Bureau Revises 2004 and 2005 Health Insurance Coverage Estimates." www.census.gov/Press-Release/www/releases/archives/health_care_insurance/009789.html.

34. K. Dychtwald, *Age Power: How the Twenty-first Century Will Be Ruled by the New Old* (New York: Tarcher/Putnam, 1999).

35. A. Lusardi and O. Mitchell, "Baby Boomer Retirement Security: The Roles of Planning, Financial Literacy and Housing Wealth," report prepared for Michigan Retirement Research Center and the Social Security Administration and presented at the University of Rochester, April 21–22, 2006.

36. See General Accountability Office (GAO), "Baby Boom Generation: Retirement of Baby Boom Generation Is Unlikely to Precipitate Dramatic Decline in Market Returns, But Broader Risks Threaten Retirement Security" (2006), for an analysis of baby boomer asset-use forecasts. www.gao.gov/highlights/d06718high.pdf.

37. C. C. Mann, "The Coming Death Shortage," *Atlantic Monthly* 295, no. 4 (2005): 92–102.

38. U.S. Census Bureau, "Current Population Survey, Annual Social and Economic Supplement" (2003). www.bls.census.gov/cps/asec/sdata.htm.

39. AARP/RoperASW, "Staying Ahead of the Curve, 2003: The AARP Working in Retirement Study" (2003). http://assets.aarp.org/rgcenter/econ/multiwork_2003.pdf.

40. J. Rowe and R. Kahn, *Successful Aging* (New York: Dell Publishing, 1998), p. 171.

41. Demographers and marketers differ on when the "echo boom" started and if it has ended. Some date the start of the "echo boom" as commencing between 1982 and 1986, and ending in the mid 90s when births peaked.

Even this narrow range, of only twelve years, produced 74 million new children, almost as large a birth cohort as the original baby boom. For purposes of this book, the "echo" began when birth numbers began rising out of their mid-1970's trough, and continues to the present.

42. J. S. Passel and R. Suro, "Rise, Peak, and Decline: Trends in U.S. Immigration, 1992–2004" (Washington, D.C., 2005). http://pewhispanic.org/files/reports/53.pdf.

43. National Center for Health Statistics, "Chartbook on Trends in the Health of Americans" (2006), fig. 1-37, p. 91. www.cdc.gov/nchs/data/hus/hus06.pdf.

44. "U.S. Population Reaches 300 Million," *Wall Street Journal,* October 17, 2006.

Three • Living to Work

1. "History of the GI Bill." www.gibill.va.gov/education/GI_Bill.htm.

2. J. E. Kwoka and C. M. Snyder, "Dynamic Adjustment in the Higher Education Industry, 1955–1997," *Review of Industrial Organization* 24, no. 4 (2003): 355–78.

3. T. Caplow, L. Hicks, and B. Wattenberg, *The First Measured Century: An Illustrated Guide to Trends in America, 1900–2000* (Washington, D.C.: American Enterprise Institute, 2001).

4. C. Conte and A. R. Karr, "An Outline of the U.S. Economy," U.S. Information Agency (2001). http://usinfo.state.gov/products/pubs/oecon/.

5. Bureau of Labor Statistics, "Employee Tenure in 2004." www.bls.gov/news.release/tenure.nr0.htm.

6. J. Schachter, "Why People Move: Exploring the March 2000 Current Population Survey," Current Population Reports, U.S. Census Bureau (2001). www .census.gov/prod/2001pubs/p23-204.pdf.

7. S. Poulos and D. Smith Nightingale, "Employment and Training Policy Implications of the Aging Baby Boom Generation" (Washington, D.C.: Urban Institute, 1997). www.urban.org/urlprint.cfm?ID=6558#char.

8. C. Goldin, "The Long Road to the Fast Track: Career and Family," National Bureau of Economic Research, Working Paper 10331 (Cambridge, Mass., 2004).

9. W. H. Frey, "Institute Review: Boomers in the 'Burbs," Milken Institute Review, no. 2 (2000): 85–91.

10. D. Brooks, Bobos in Paradise: The New Upper Class and How They Got There (New York: Touchstone Books, 2000), p. 135.

11. "U.S. Job Satisfaction Keeps Falling, the Conference Board Reports Today," Conference Board, 2005 www.conference-board.org/utilities/pressDetail .cfm?press_ID=2582.

12. B. Hagenbaugh, "U.S. Manufacturing Jobs Fading Away Fast," USA Today, December 12, 2002.

13. "Union Members in 2006," Bureau of Labor Statistics USDL 07-0113. www.bls.gov/news.release/pdf/union2.pdf.

14. P. Coy, "Old, Smart, Productive," Business Week, June 27, 2005, p. 78.

15. PBGC Public Affairs. "Companies Report a Record $353.7 Billion Pension Shortfall in Latest Filings with PBGC." www.pbgc.gov/media/news-archive/ 2005/pr05-48.html.

16. MedPac Survey of Employer-Sponsored Health Benefits, 2004, p. 64. www.medpac.gov/publications/congressional_reports/june05databookSec6.pdf.

17. C. Milner, "Re-visioning Retirement," Journal on Active Aging, July–August 2003, p. 31.

18. J. K. Morris, D. G. Cook, and A. G. Shaper, "Loss of Employment and Mortality," British Medical Journal 308, no. 6937 (1994): 1135–39.

19. American Association of Suicidology, "Elderly Suicide Fact Sheet" (2002). www.211bigbend.org/hotlines/suicide/SuicideandtheElderly.pdf.

20. AIG SunAmerica/Harris Interactive, "Revisioning Retirement" (2002). www.re-visioningretirement.com/PDF/completesurvey.pdf.

21. S. Zapolsky, "Baby Boomers Envision Retirement II: Survey of Baby Boomers' Expectations for Retirement" (Washington, D.C.: AARP, 2004).

22. Pew Research Center, "Working after Retirement: The Gap between Expectations and Reality" (2006). http://pewresearch.org/assets/social/pdf/ Retirement.pdf.

23. Author's analysis of P. F. Adams and P. M. Barnes, "Summary Health Statistics for the U.S. Population: National Health Interview Survey, 2004," National Center for Health Statistics, Vital Health Statistics, series 10, no. 229 (2006). www.cdc.gov/nchs/data/series/sr_10/sr10_229.pdf.

24. AARP/RoperASW, "Staying Ahead of the Curve 2003: The AARP Working in Retirement Study" (2003). http://assets.aarp.org/rgcenter/econ/multi work_2003.pdf.

25. AARP, "Boomers Envision Retirement."

26. K. Dychtwald, *The Age Wave: How The Most Important Trend of Our Time Can Change Your Future* (New York: Bantam Books, 1990).

27. AARP, "Staying Ahead of the Curve."

28. J. Zissimopolous and L. Karoly, "Work and Wellbeing among the Self-Employed at Older Ages," AARP Public Policy Institute (Washington, D.C.: AARP, 2007).

29. Bureau of Labor Statistics reported in J. B. Quinn, "Your Retirement: How to Land on Your Feet," *Newsweek*, February 14, 2005, p. 50.

30. S. Moffett, "Senior Moment: Fast-Aging Japan Keeps Its Elders on the Job Longer," *Wall Street Journal*, June 15, 2005.

31. B. Butrica and C. Uccello, "How Will Boomers Fare at Retirement?" Urban Institute (2004). www.urban.org/UploadedPDF/900767_boomers_retire ment.pdf.

32. R. B. Avery and M. S. Rendall, "Estimating the Size and Distribution of Baby Boomers' Prospective Inheritances," American Statistical Association, *Proceedings of the Social Statistics Section* (1993): 11–19.

33. K. Dychtwald, *Workforce Crisis* (Boston: Harvard Business School Press, 2006).

34. Bureau of Labor Statistics, "Current Population Survey, 2007," table A-4: Employment Status of the Civilian Population 25 Years and Over by Educational Attainment. www.bls.gov/webapps.legacy/cpsatab4.htm.

35. A. Carnevale and D. Desrochers, "Why Learning: The Value of Higher Education to Society and the Individual," ch. 5, *Keeping America's Promise*, Education Commission of the States (2004). www.ecs.org/ecsmain.asp?page=/html/educa tionissues/ECSStateNotes.asp.

36. J. C. Mihm, "Human Capital: Federal Workforce Challenges," Testimony before the Subcommittee on Financial Services and General Government, Committee on Appropriations, House of Representatives, March 6, 2007.

37. *Managing Federal Recruitment: Issues, Insights, and Illustrations*, a report to the President and the Congress of the United States by the U.S. Merit Systems Protection Board (2004).

38. General Accounting Office, "FAA Needs to Better Prepare for Impending Wave of Controller Attrition" (2002). www.gao.gov/new.items/d02591.pdf.

39. Association of State and Territorial Health Officials, "State Public Health Employee Worker Shortage Report: A Civil Service Recruitment and Retention Crisis," December 2003. www.astho.org/pubs/Workforce-Survey-Report-2.pdf.

40. U.S. Department of Education, National Center for Education Statistics, Schools and Staffing Survey, "Public Teacher Questionnaire," "Charter Teacher

Questionnaire," and "Private Teacher Questionnaire," 1999–2000. http://nces
.ed.gov/pubsearch/pubsinfo.asp?pubid=2002313.

41. National Center for Education Information, "Profile of Teachers in the US 2005" (2005). www/ncei.com/Poto5PRESSREL3.htm.

42. M. Mandel, "What's Really Propping up the Economy," *Business Week*, September 25, 2006.

43. L. Briggs, "AORN 2000 Member/Nonmember Needs Assessment Results," *AORN Journal* 72 (2000): 586–90.

44. Ibid.

45. J. C. Goldsmith and N. Kaufman, "Between a Rock and a Hard Place: Physician Markets Create New Strategic Problems for Hospital," *COR Healthcare Market Strategist* (November 2004): 20–24.

46. D. K. Foot, R. P. Lewis, T. A. Pearson, and G. A. Beller, "Demographics and Cardiology, 1950–2050," *Journal of the American College of Cardiology* 35, no. 4 (2000): 1067–81.

47. Physician Compensation Report, "General Surgery Starts to See Shortage of Residents Due to Lifestyle, Pay Issues," April 2002. www.findarticles.com/p/articles/mi_m0FBW/is_4_3/ai_84408455.

48. Council on Graduate Medical Education, "Physician Workforce Policy Guidelines for the United States, 2000–2020," Sixteenth Report (2005). www.cogme.gov/16.pdf.

49. Association of American Medical Colleges, "The Physician Workforce: Position Statement" (2005). www.aamc.org/workforce/12704workforce.pdf.

50. Statement of C. Eugene Steuerle, Senior Fellow, Urban Institute, Codirector, Tax Policy Center, and Columnist, *Tax Notes Magazine*, Testimony before the House Committee on Ways and Means, May 12, 2005.

51. R. Florida, *Flight of the Creative Class: The New Global Competition for Talent* (New York: Harper Business, 2005), pp. 11–13.

Four • Healthy Aging

1. S. Moore and J. L. Simon, "The Greatest Century That Ever Was: Twenty-five Miraculous Trends of the Past 100 Years," *Policy Analysis*, no. 364 (Washington, D.C.: Cato Institute, 1999).

2. J. Oeppen and J. W. Vaupel, "Broken Limits to Life Expectancy," *Science* 296, no. 5570 (2002): 1029–31.

3. E. M. Gruenberg, "The Failures of Success," *Milbank Memorial Fund Quarterly* 55, no. 1 (1977): 3–24.

4. J. F. Fries, "Aging, Natural Death and the Compression of Morbidity," *New England Journal of Medicine* 303, no. 3 (1980): 130–35.

5. K. G. Manton, X. Gu, and V. Lamb, "Change in Chronic Disability from 1982 to 2004/2005 as Measured by Long Term Changes in Function and Health

in the U.S. Elderly Population," *PNAS* 103, no. 48 (2006): 18374–79. www.pnas
.org/cgi/doi/10.1073/pnas.0608483103.

6. Ibid.

7. J. P. Leigh and J. F. Fries, "Education, Gender and the Compression of
Morbidity," *International Journal of Aging and Human Development* 39, no. 3
(1994): 233–46.

8. L. D. Kubzansky et al., "Is Educational Attainment Associated with Shared
Determinants of Health in the Elderly? Findings from the MacArthur Studies of
Successful Aging," *American Psychosomatic Society* 60, no. 5 (1998): 578–85.

9. J. C. Goldsmith, "Technologies and the Boundaries of the Hospital: Three
Emerging Technologies," *Health Affairs* 23, no. 6 (2004): 149–56.

10. S. J. Shieh and J. P. Vacanti, "State-of-the-Art Tissue Engineering: From
Tissue Engineering to Organ Building," *Surgery* 137, no. 1 (2005): 1–7; M. Papadaki
"Cellular/Tissue Engineering," *Engineering in Medicine and Biology IEEE* 23, no. 5
(2004): 84–90; D. J. Mooney and A. G. Mikos, "Growing New Organs," *Scientific
American* 280, no. 4 (1999): 60–65; G. Q. Daley, M. A. Goodell, and E. Y. Snyder,
"Realistic Prospects for Stem Cell Therapeutics," *Hematology* 1 (2003): 398–418.

11. S. Cohen and J. Leor, "Rebuilding Broken Hearts," *Scientific American* 291,
no. 5 (2004): 45–52.

12. J. H. Herndon, "The Future of Orthopaedics," *American Academy of Orthopedic Surgeons Bulletin* 52, no. 3 (2004). www2.aaos.org/aaos/archives/bulletin/
jun04/fline3.htm; American Society of Plastic Surgeons, "2000/2005/2006 National Plastic Surgery Statistics: Cosmetic and Reconstructive Procedure Trends."
www.plasticsurgery.org/media/statistics/loader.cfrm?url=/commonspot/security/
getfile.cfm&PageID=23628.

13. T. Pearson, "The Prevention of Cardiovascular Disease: Have We Really
Made Progress?" *Health Affairs* 26, no. 1 (2007): 49–60.

14. K. Safavi, Chief Medical Officer, Solucient, "By the Numbers: Emerging
Trends in Hospital Services," presentation to Forum for Healthcare Strategists,
Las Vegas, Nev., May 2006.

15. S. Dominus, "Life in the Age of Old, Old Age," *New York Times Magazine*,
February 22, 2004.

16. U.S. Census Bureau, "Centenarians in the United States," Current Population Reports, Special Studies, July 1999. www.census.gov/prod/99/pubs/p23-
199pdf.

17. M. J. Hall, "2001 National Hospital Discharge Survey," Centers for Disease
Control and Prevention, no. 332 (2003). www.cdc.gov/hchs/data/ad/ad332.pdf.

18. C. C. Mann, "The Coming Death Shortage," *Atlantic Monthly* 295, no. 4
(2005): 92–102.

19. D. Goldman, B. Shang, et al., "Consequences of Health Trends and Medical Innovation for the Future Elderly," *Health Affairs* (Web Exclusive) 24, no. 2
(2005): W5, R5–17.

20. This is why we urgently need a small but powerful federal agency to weigh the value of technological innovation in medicine, and inform coverage and payment decisions. Modeling the cost side of the technology equation is necessary but not sufficient for making policy. See G. Wilensky, "Developing a Center for Comparative Effectiveness Information," *Health Affairs* 25, no. 1 (2006): 174–85, and the discussion papers following.

21. D. Cutler, "The Potential for Cost Savings in Medicare's Future," *Health Affairs* (Web Exclusive) 24, no. 2 (2005): W5, R77–80.

22. J. Lubitz et al., "Health, Life Expectancy and Health Care Spending among the Elderly," *New England Journal of Medicine* 349, no. 11 (2003): 1054.

23. S. Calfo, J. Smith, and M. Zezza, "Last Year of Life Study," September 17, 2004. www.cms.hhs.gov/statistics/lyol/default.asp.

24. J. Rowe and R. Kahn, *Successful Aging* (New York: Dell Publishing, 1998).

25. S. J. Olshansky, D. Passaro, R. Hershow, et al., "A Potential Decline in Life Expectancy in the United States in the Twenty-first Century," *New England Journal of Medicine* 352, no. 11 (2005): 1138–45.

26. K. E. Thorpe et al., "The Impact of Obesity on Rising Medical Spending," *Health Affairs* (Web Exclusive) (2004): W4, 480–86.

27. W. Gibbs, "Obesity: An Overblown Epidemic?" *Scientific American* 292, no. 6 (2005): 70–77.

28. K. M. Flegal et al., "Excess Deaths Associated with Underweight, Overweight, and Obesity," *Journal of the American Medical Association* 293, no. 15 (2005): 1861–67.

29. D. Lakdawalla, D. Goldman, and B. Shang, "The Health and Cost Consequences of Obesity among the Future Elderly," *Health Affairs* (Web Exclusive) 24, no. 2 (2005): W5, R31–41.

30. R. Robinson, "Alzheimer's Disease," *Gale Encyclopedia of Medicine* (Gale Research, 1999).

31. L. E. Hebert et al., "Alzheimer Disease in the U.S. Population: Prevalence Estimates Using the 2000 Census," *Archives of Neurology* 60, no. 8 (2003): 1119–22.

32. See comment by Fernando Pico, Julien Labreuche, Pierre-Jean Touboul, Didier Leys, and Pierre Amarenco for the GENIC Investigators, "Intracranial Arterial Dolichoectasia and Small-Vessel Disease in Stroke Patients," *Annals of Neurology* 57, no. 4, (2005): 472–79.

33. J. Caballero and M. Hahata, "Do Statins Slow Down Alzheimer's Disease?" *Journal of Clinical Pharmacy and Therapeutics* 29, no. 3 (2004): 209–13.

34. B. J. Soldo, O. B. Mitchell, et al., "Cross-Cohort Differences in Health on the Verge of Retirement," University of Pennsylvania, Population Aging Research Center, Working Paper Series 0-13, September 2006.

Five • Encouraging Work in Later Life

1. R. Reich, *Work of Nations: Preparing Ourselves for Twenty-first Century Capitalism* (New York: A. A. Knopf, 1991).

2. R. Florida, *The Rise of the Creative Class* (New York: Basic Books, 2002).

3. World Intellectual Property Organization, Statistical Data Query: PCT International Applications (2007). www.wipo.int/ipstatsdb/en/stats.jsp.

4. National Science Foundation, "Science and Engineering Indicators, 2004," appendix table 6-11. www.nsf.gov/statistics/seind04.

5. M. Heylin, "Science Is Becoming Truly Worldwide," *Chemical and Engineering News* 82, no. 24 (2004): 38–41.

6. "What's Really Propping Up the Economy," *Business Week,* September 25, 2006, pp. 55–62.

7. U.S. Congress, House of Representatives, Report by the House Small Business Committee, "Small Business Index, 2005, First Quarter," June 2005.

8. M. Wolk, "Small Business Having a Big Impact on Jobs," February 3, 2004, MSNBC.com.

9. J. A. Zoltan and C. Armington, "Endogenous Growth and Entrepreneurial Activity in Cities," U.S. Department of Commerce, Bureau of the Census, Center for Economic Studies, Working Paper (Washington, D.C., 2003).

10. U.S. Census Bureau, Department of Commerce, Washington, D.C., "Nonemployer Statistics, 2003," October 2005. www.census.gov/Press-Release/www/releases/acrhives/business_ownership/005784.html.

11. "Telework Trending Upward, Survey Says," WorldatWork press release, September 21, 2007. www.workingfromanywhere.org/news/pr020707.html.

12. J. P. Mello, "Home-Sourcing vs. Offshoring," January 26, 2005, CFO.com.

13. Fox News, "Telemarketing Goes Home," May 29, 2005, Foxnews.com.

14. M. Naumann, "Reporter Touts Benefits of Telecommuting" *San Jose Mercury News*, September 9, 2007.

15. E. Safirova and M. Walls, Resources for the Future, "What Have We Learned from a Recent Survey of Teleworkers? Evaluating the 2002 Southern California Association of Governments Survey," Discussion Paper 04-43 (Washington, D.C., 2004). www.rff.org/documents/RFF-DP-04-43.pdf.

16. M. J. Breslow et al., "Effect of an ICU Telemedicine Program on Clinical and Economic Outcomes," *Critical Care Medicine* 32, no. 1 (2004): 31–38.

17. R. G. Penner, P. Perun, and E. Steuerle, "Legal and Institutional Impediments to Partial Retirement and Part-time Work by Older Workers," Working Paper (Washington, D.C.: Urban Institute Press, 2002).

18. Age Discrimination in Employment Act of 1967, Pub. L. No. 90-202, 81 Stat. 602 (December 15, 1967), codified as Chapter 14 of Title 29 of the United States Code, 29 U.S.C. §621 through 29 U.S.C. §634 (ADEA).

19. B. L. Atencio et al., "Nurse Retention: Is It Worth It?" *Nursing Economics* 21, no. 6 (2003): 262–68.

20. HSM Group, Ltd., "Acute Care Hospital Survey of RN Vacancy and Turnover Rates in 2000," *Journal of Nursing Administration* 32, no. 9 (200): 437–39.

21. "The Business Case for Workers Age 50+," Towers Perrin (2005). www .aarp.org/research/work/employment/workers_fifty_plus.html.

22. R. Stouffer, "Health Care Temps in Big Demand," *Pittsburgh Tribune Review,* March 9, 2005.

23. A. S. McCampbell, "Benefits Achieved through Alternative Work Schedules," *Human Resource Planning* 19, no. 3 (1996). www.allbusiness.com/human-resources/583809-1.html.

24. J. R. Marshall et al., "Job Sharing and the Clinical Nurse Specialist Role," *Nursing Management* 24, no. 11 (1993): 78–80.

25. M. Freudenheim, "More Help Wanted: Older Workers Please Apply," *New York Times,* March 23, 2005.

26. K. Dychtwald, *Workforce Crisis* (Boston: Harvard Business School Press, 2006), p. 79.

27. Dawn Malone, Bon Secours Health System-Richmond, Human Resources, personal communication, February 28, 2007.

28. "Phased Retirement: IRS Regulations Leave Hurdles to be Overcome," Employment Policy Foundation, Washington, D.C., March 31, 2005.

29. W. M. Mercer, "Capitalizing on an Aging Workforce: Phased Retirement and Other Options," William Mercer and Company, April 2001.

30. S. F. Gale, "Phased Retirement," *Workforce Management* (2003). www .workforce.com/section/02/feature/23/47/31/.

31. Penner, Perun, and Steuerle, "Legal and Institutional Impediments."

32. R. Penner et al., "Letting Older Workers Work," Urban Institute, The Retirement Project, Brief Series no. 1 (Washington, D.C., July 2003).

33. Ibid.

34. John Bertko, Humana actuary, personal communication, March 18, 2005.

35. Health Care Policy Roundtable, "First Wave of Large Employers Opens the Door to Affordable Health Insurance for More than 1 Million Workers" (2005). www.hcpr.org/news/news_story.asp?ID=2251.

36. "Freelancers of the World, Unite!" *Economist,* November 9, 2006. Also, personal communication, Sara Horowitz, Working Today, September 20, 2007. See their website, www.freelancersunion.org, for a listing of its offerings.

37. E. Porter, "Coming Soon: The Vanishing Work Force," *New York Times,* August 29, 2004.

38. L. E. Burman and J. Gruber, "Tax Credits for Health Insurance," Urban-Brookings Tax Policy Center (2005). www.taxpolicycenter.org/publications/url .cfm?ID=311189.

39. For a description of Wyden's approach, see L. Meckler, "How Plans to Ex-

pand Health Coverage Could Affect Insured," *Wall Street Journal,* February 6, 2007.

40. V. R. Fuchs and E. J. Emanuel, "Health Care Reform: Why? What? When?" *Health Affairs* 24, no. 6 (2005): 1399–1414.

41. M. W. Serafini, "The Mass.-ter Plan," *National Journal* 38, no. 22 (2006). http://nationaljournal.com/pubs/nj/.

42. L. Belkin, "When Whippersnappers and Geezers Collide," *New York Times,* July 26, 2007.

43. Dychtwald, *Workforce Crisis.*

44. W. A. Achenbaum, *Social Security: Visions and Revisions,* A Twentieth Century Fund Study (Cambridge: Cambridge University Press, 1986), pp. 192–93.

45. Microsoft, "Digital Workstyle: The New World of Work" (2005). http://download.microsoft.com/download/B/E/4/BE40F0BC-434B-487C-B788-20052D75A3EC/NewWorldofWorkWP.doc.

46. P. Coy, "Old, Smart, Productive," *Business Week,* June 27, 2005, p. 81.

47. C. E. Steuerle, "Social Security and the Trustees Report: Statement before the Committee on the Budget," U.S. House of Representatives, June 19, 2002.

48. B. Butirca, K. Smith, and E. Steurle, "Working for a Good Retirement," Urban Institute Retirement Project, Discussion Paper 06-03 (Washington, D.C., 2006).

Six • Medicare

1. OECD, National Accounts Database (2006). www.oecd.org/dataoecd/48/4/37867909.pdf.

2. J. Poisal, C. Truffer, S. Smith, et al., 2007. "Health Spending Projections through 2016: Modest Changes Obscure Part D's Impact," *Health Affairs* (Web Exclusive) (2007): W248. www.healthaffairs.org/cgi/reprint/26/2/W<->242.

3. L. J. Kotlikoff and S. Burns, *The Coming Generational Storm: What You Need to Know about America's Economic Future* (Cambridge, Mass.: MIT Press, 2004), p. 51.

4. In 2007 the Office of the Actuary for the Centers for Medicare and Medicaid Services reduced its ten-year health care cost growth forecast from 7.3 percent per year to 6.9 percent per year. The difference between these two forecasts, applied to Medicare alone, over a fifty-year period, using FY2006 actual spending as the base, is $2.4 trillion (author's calculation).

5. R. H. Brook, "Perspectives on Medicare: Medicare Quality and Getting Older: A Personal Essay," *Health Affairs* 14, no. 4 (1995): 73–81.

6. T. Bodenheimer, R. A. Berenson, et al., "The Primary Care-Specialty Income Gap: Why It Matters," *Annals of Internal Medicine* 146, no. 4 (2007): 301–6.

7. See Christine Cassel's *Medicare Matters: What Geriatric Medicine Can Teach American Health Care* (Berkeley: University of California Press, 2005), for a discussion of Medicare's inadequate focus on chronic disease.

8. "A Profile of Caregiving in American, 2nd ed.," *Pfizer Journal* 9, no. 4 (2005): 9.

9. K. Dychtwald, *Age Power: How the Twenty-first Century Will Be Ruled by the New Old* (New York: Tarcher/Penguin, 1999), p. 146.

10. "Fear of Litigation Study," conducted by Harris Interactive, April 11, 2002. http://cgood.org/assets/attachments/68.pdf. See also M. Mello et al., "Caring for Patients in a Malpractice Crisis: Physician Satisfaction and the Quality of Care," *Health Affairs* 23, no. 4, 42–53.

11. Statement of Glenn M. Hackbarth, Chairman, Medicare Payment Advisory Commission, Testimony before the Subcommittee on Health of the House Committee on Ways and Means, May 1, 2003.

12. Henry J. Kaiser Family Foundation, "Medicare Fact Sheet: The Medicare Prescription Drug Benefit" (2007). www.kff.org/medicare/upload/7044-06.pdf.

13. M. Moon, "Getting It Right: Issues for Medicare Reform," Testimony of Marilyn Moon, Urban Institute, prepared for Senate Finance Committee, June 6, 2003. Original cost estimates came from Fidelity Corp.

14. M. Fruedenheim, "Fewer Employers Totally Cover Health Premiums," *New York Times,* March 23, 2005.

15. J. Wennberg, et al., "Chronic Illness and the Problem of Supply-Sensitive Care," *Dartmouth Atlas of Health Care* (2006). www.dartmouthatlas.org/atlases/2006_Chronic_Care_Atlas.pdf.

16. C. Boccuti, M. Moon, and K. Dowling, "Policy Brief: Chronic Conditions and Disabilities; Trends and Issues for Private Drug Plans," Commonwealth Fund (2003). www.commonwealthfund.org/publications/publications_show.htm?doc_id=221565.

17. J. C. Goldsmith, *Digital Medicine* (Chicago: Health Administration Press, 2003).

18. J. H. Gurwitz et al., "Incidence and Prevalence of Adverse Drug Events among Older Persons in the Ambulatory Setting," *Journal of the American Medical Association* 289, no. 9 (2003): 1107–16.

19. University of Massachusetts Medical School, "Adverse Drug Events among Older Persons in the Outpatient Setting Are Common and Preventable" (2003). www.umassmed.edu/pap/news/2003/03_04_03.cfm.

20. MedPac, "A Databook: Healthcare Spending and the Medicare Program" (2006). www.medpac.gov/publications/congressional_reports/Jun06DataBook_Entire_report.pdf.

21. Merritt, Hawkins & Associates. "2004 Survey of Physicians 50–65 Years Old," Summary Report. www.merritthawkins.com/pdf/2004_physician50_survey.pdf.

22. Ibid.

23. For a superb discussion of the history and politics of Medicare's payment changes, see R. Mayes and R. Berenson, *Medicare Prospective Payment and the Shaping of U.S. Health Care* (Baltimore: Johns Hopkins University Press, 2007).

24. K. Davis, M. Moon, et al., "Medicare Extra: A Comprehensive Benefit Option for Medicare Beneficiaries," *Health Affairs* (Web Exclusive) (October 2005): W5, 442–53.

25. See A. H. Goroll, R. A. Berenson, et al. 2007. "Fundamental Reform of Payment for Adult Primary Care: Comprehensive Payment for Comprehensive Care," *Journal of General Internal Medicine*, 22(3): 410–15, for a detailed discussion of this approach.

26. See C. Sia, T. Tonniges, et al. 2004, "A History of the Medical Home Concept," *Pediatrics* 113, no. 4 (2004): 1473–78, for a comprehensive review of this evolving idea.

27. Kaiser Family Foundation, "Health Insurance Coverage in America: 2005 Data Update," November 2006. www.kff.org/uninsured/upload/2005Data Update.pdf.

28. J. M. McWilliams, E. Meara, A. Zaslavsky, and J. Ayanian, "Use of Health Services by Previously Uninsured Medicare Beneficiaries," *New England Journal of Medicine* 357, no. 2 (2007): 150.

29. Cassel, *Medicare Matters*, p. 109.

30. McWilliams, Meara, Zaslavsky, and Ayanian, "Use of Health Services by Previously Uninsured Medicare Beneficiaries."

31. W. A. Achenbaum, *Older Americans, Vital Communities: A Bold Vision for Societal Aging* (Baltimore: Johns Hopkins University Press, 2005), p. 81.

32. Ibid.

33. V. Villagra and T. Ahmed, "Effectiveness of a Disease Management Program for Patients with Diabetes," *Health Affairs* 23, no. 4 (2004): 255–66; F. A. McAlister, F. M. E. Lawson, et al., "A Systematic Review of Randomized Trials of Disease Management Programs in Heart Failure," *American Journal of Medicine* 10 (2001): 378–84.

Seven • Social Security Reform

1. L. J. Kotlikoff and S. Burns, *The Coming Generational Storm: What You Need to Know about America's Economic Future* (Cambridge, Mass.: MIT Press, 2004), p. 51.

2. See "Bush's Plan for Social Security," February 2, 2005, CNNMoney.com. http://money.cnn.com/2005/02/02/retirement/stofunion_socsec/index.htm, for a summary of key points of this proposal.

3. B. Basler, "Changing Social Security: Will Young People Go for It?" *AARP Bulletin Online* (2005). www.aarp.org/bulletin/socialsec/ss_younggen.html.

4. Economic Policy Institute, "Social Security; Facts at a Glance" (2005). www.epinet.org/content.cfm/issueguide_socialsecurityfacts.

5. C. Davies et al., "A Changing Political Landscape as One Generation Replaces Another" (Washington, D.C.: AARP, 2004), p. 9.

6. Social Security Administration Online, "Actuarial Publications: Trust Fund Data." www.ssa.gov/OACT/STATS/table 4a1./html. Data are for the year 2006, as of February 2007.

7. See A. Sloan, "Social Security: A Daring Leap," *Newsweek*, February 14, 2005, pp. 41–44, for a comprehensible discussion of the Social Security funding problem.

8. "Getting the Public to Listen," Democracy Corps, Washington, D.C., February 28, 2007.

9. E. Steuerle, "2005 Lifetime Medicare Tables," and "2005 Lifetime SS Tables" (Washington, D.C.: Urban Institute, 2005).

10. J. Gohkale and K. Smetters, "Fiscal and General Imbalances: New Budget Measures for New Budget Priorities," Federal Reserve Bank of Cleveland, Policy Discussion Paper, March 2002.

11. Kotlikoff and Burns take a different and more intriguing approach. They essentially shut down the pension part of Social Security (leaving the survivor and disability part intact). They replace most of the current Social Security tax with a temporary, declining national sales tax to pay accrued Social Security benefits for current retirees, as well as the accumulated benefits earned by current workers. Instead of paying a Social Security payroll tax going forward, workers would pay an equivalent amount into private accounts invested in a global index fund indexed to stocks, bonds, and real estate. It is a creative, if somewhat scary, solution, akin to putting a heart bypass surgery patient on the heart-lung pump before replacing his occluded arteries.

12. C. Isidore, "The Zero Savings Problem," CNN/Money (2005). http://money.cnn.com/2005/08/02/news/economy/savings/?cnn=yes.

13. G. Mermin, "Reforming Social Security through Price and Progressive Price Indexing," Urban Institute (2005). www.urban.org/UploadedPDF/900903_reforming_ss.pdf.

14. M. Favreault, G. Mermin, et al., "Minimum Benefits in Social Security Could Reduce Aged Poverty," Urban Institute, The Retirement Project, no. 11 (Washington, D.C., 2007).

15. Ibid.; J. Gist and K. Wu, "The Inequality of Financial Wealth among Boomers," AARP Public Policy Institute Data Digest, July 2004; M. Zuckerman, "A 'Cure' Worse than the Cold," *U.S. News and World Report* (2005), www.usnews.com/usnews/opinion/articles/050131/31edit.htm.

16. G. Burtless, "Increasing the Eligibility Age for Social Security Pensions," Brookings Institution, Testimony before Senate Special Committee on Aging, July 15, 1998.

17. U.S. Government Accountability Office, "Disability Insurance; SSA Should Strengthen Its Efforts to Detect and Prevent Overpayments," Report to the Chair, Committee on Finance, U.S. Senate (2004). www.gao.gov/new.items/d04929.pdf; A. B. Krueger, "Disability Insurance Side of Social Security Raises Questions," *New York Times*, March 3, 2005.

18. Krueger, "The Disability Insurance Side of Social Security Raises Some Questions."

19. M. Moore, "Social Security Reform: Looking at the Options," National Center for Policy Analysis, no. 504 (Dallas, Tex., 2005).

20. P. R. Orszag, "Should a Lump Sum Payment Replace Social Security's Delayed Retirement Credit," Center for Retirement Research at Boston College, An Issue in Brief, no. 6 (Boston, April 2001).

21. L. Etheredge, "Three Streams, One River: A Coordinated Approach to Financing Retirement," *Health Affairs* 18, no. 1 (1999): 80–91.

22. Statement of C. Eugene Steuerle, Senior Fellow, Urban Institute, Codirector, Tax Policy Center, and Columnist, *Tax Notes Magazine,* Testimony before the House Committee on Ways and Means, May 12, 2005.

23. "A Long, Long Life," *Economist,* March 27, 2004.

24. K. Ignagni, Testimony on Long-Term Care and Medicaid: Spiraling Costs and the Need for Reform, before the U.S. House Committee on Energy and Commerce Subcommittee on Health, April 27, 2005.

25. Ideally, people should enroll in long-term care insurance earlier than age 65 (e.g., in their early to middle 50s). But half of 65-year-olds will live at least another twenty years, and those twenty years could permit some sheltering of assets for long-term care expenses through private insurance.

26. Etheredge, "Three Streams, One River."

Eight • What We Need to Do

1. T. L. Friedman, *The World Is Flat* (New York: Farrar, Straus and Giroux, 2005).

2. D. Gross, "Cigarettes, Taxes and Thin French Women," *New York Times,* July 24, 2005.

3. P. Longman, "The Best Care Anywhere," *Washington Monthly,* January–February 2005. www.washingtonmonthly.com/features/2005/0501.longman .html; J. B. Perlin, R. M. Kolodner, and R. H. Roswell, "The Veterans Health Administration: Quality, Value, Accountability, and Information as Transforming Strategies for Patient-Centered Care," *American Journal of Managed Care* 10, no. 2 (2004): 828–36.

4. Interagency Council on the Homeless, "The Forgotten Americans: Homelessness; Programs and the People They Serve," National Survey of Homeless Assistance Providers and Clients, National Coalition for Homeless Veterans, Washington, D.C. (1999).

5. "Returning to the Nest," *Baltimore Sun,* February 29, 2004. www.theeagle .com/businesstechnology/022904returnnest.htm; "Boomerang Kids Keep Coming Home," CBS Evening News, January 9, 2004, www.cbsnews.com/stories/2004/01/08/eveningnews/main/592186.shtml.

6. J. Deparle, *American Dream* (New York: Penguin Group, 2004).

7. Internal Revenue Service, "EITC Information and Resources for Individuals." www.irs.gov/individuals/article/0,,id=96406,00.html.

8. R. V. Burkhauser and J. F. Quinn, "Implementing Pro-Work Policies for Older Americans in the Twenty-first Century," paper prepared for the U.S. Senate Subcommittee on Aging, Forum on Older Workers (1997).

Nine • What Baby Boomers Should Do for Themselves

1. R. M. Henig, "Will We Ever Arrive at the Good Death?" *New York Times Magazine*, August 7, 2005, pp. 26–36, 40, 68.

2. See Judith Turiel's passionate and useful treatise on these issues. J. Turiel, *Our Parents, Ourselves* (Berkeley: University of California Press, 2005).

3. S. Beider, "An Ethical Argument for Integrated Palliative Care," *Evidence-Based Complementary Alternative Medicine* 2, no. 2 (2005): 227–31.

4. "High Court Upholds Oregon Assisted-Suicide Law," MSNBC, January 18, 2006. www.msnbc.msn.com/id/10891536.

5. U.S. Department of Health and Human Services, "Physical Activity and Health: A Report of the Surgeon General" (Atlanta: U.S. Department of Health and Human Services, Centers for Disease Control and Prevention, National Center for Chronic Disease Prevention and Health Promotion, 1996).

6. Cynthia Kenyon, University of California, San Francisco, personal communication, May 3, 2005.

7. L. Eisenberg, *The Number: A Completely Different Way to Think about the Rest of Your Life* (New York: Free Press, 2006).

Conclusion

1. "The Entitlement Panic," editorial, *Wall Street Journal*, August 22, 2006.

Index

AARP, xiii, 30
abortion rights, 18–19, 46
Achenbaum, W. A., 98, 159
Age Discrimination in Employment Act
   (ADEA), 88, 89, 90, 92
air traffic controllers, 59
Alzheimer's disease, 76–78
Arab oil embargo, 12
automobiles, 13

baby boomers: attitudes toward Medicare,
   131; attitudes toward Social Security, 152–
   53; and chronic illnesses, 162–63; cultural divisions among, 17–18; differing
   trajectories of, 1–8, 52–55, 154–66; diversity of, 52–55; early years of, 9; education
   levels of, 11, 66–67; and end-of-life decisions, 173–74; and entitlement programs,
   32; financial difficulties of, 53–54, 158–61,
   165–66; flexible work schedules for, 90–
   93; future of, xi–xiii, 69–71, 169–77, 178–
   83; health habits of, 74, 157–58, 162;
   health of, xiv–xv, 7–8, 65–71, 78–79, 129–
   30, 171–73; and knowledge-based economy, 86–87; life expectancy of, 64–65; in
   the military, 14–15; optimism of, 22–24;
   personal growth of, 101–2; political activism of, 13–15, 30; political distrust of,
   18–20; and popular culture, 12–13; productivity of, 100; resentment toward, 17;
   retirement plans of, xiii–xiv, 87–90; self-
   perception of, 24; and social policy, xii,
   xv–xvii, 42, 166–68; as veterans, 164–65;
voting patterns of, 19–20; wealth of, 22,
   38–39, 56–57, 154–55; work as important
   to, 48–50, 52; in the work force, xiii–xiv,
   1–3, 39, 55–56, 57–59, 61–63, 80, 87–90,
   166–68, 170. *See also* Medicare; Social
   Security
Beatles, the, 13
Begala, Paul, 17
black Americans, political activism on behalf of, 14
Bon Secours Health System, 92
Brooks, David, 49
Burns, S., xi–xii, 34, 35, 36
Bush, George W., 20, 23; and Social Security reform, 133–34

cancer, 68
Capelli, Peter, 30
capital gains taxes, 156
caregivers, 61
cars, 13
Carter, Jimmy, 23
Cassel, Christine, 124
catastropharian thesis, xii–xiii; and entitlement programs, 34–36, 104; and increased life expectancy, 65, 71–72;
   problems with, 37–41
cell therapy, 68
chronic illnesses, 68; and baby boomers,
   161–62; and Medicare, 106–7
civil rights movement, 14, 18–19
Clapton, Eric, 13
Clinton, Bill, 19, 23

About the Author

Jeff Goldsmith is an author, lecturer, and strategy consultant. He is president of Health Futures, Inc., and an associate professor of public health sciences at the University of Virginia. He has taught at the University of Chicago's Graduate School of Business and the Wharton School at the University of Pennsylvania. After obtaining his doctorate in sociology from the University of Chicago in 1973, he worked for the governor of Illinois and the dean of the School of Medicine at the University of Chicago. For more than thirty years he has worked in health care management and policy. He lives at Ricochet Farm, near Charlottesville, Virginia.